GAMES

Gym Activties Made Easy & Simple

Jim Eagan   B.S., M.S.

Tom Caione   B.S., M.S., P.D.

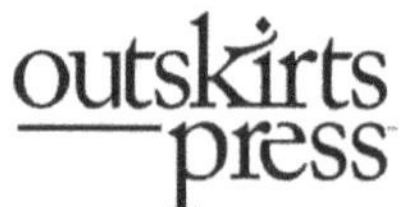

Illustration Credits

Interior Images © Copyright 2000-2020 Dreamstime.
All rights reserved - used with permission.

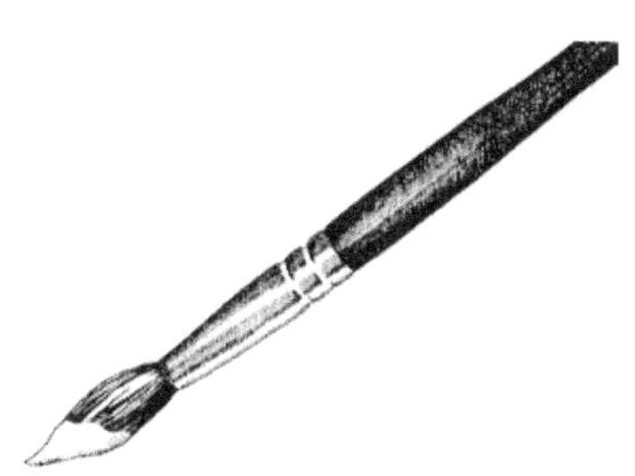

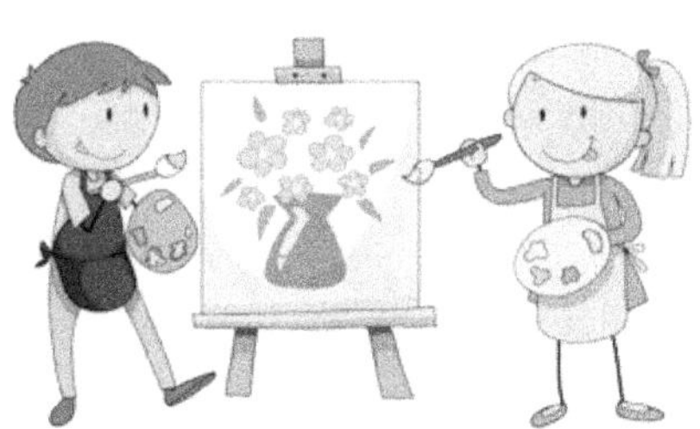

Introduction

We first got the idea for this book of activities during a discussion that Jim Eagan and I were having about the state of "Elementary Physical Education" in American Schools today. After reading literally hundreds of publications with several great ideas, we found that many of these ideas were totally unrealistic in today's world of **large class sizes, inadequate facilities, and limited budgets.**   Add to this a preponderance of pre-kindergarten students, and the need to provide classroom teachers with "common planning time", and you have in many cases, an impossible learning situation for elementary physical education students.

School Administrator's (of which I was one), are being forced to schedule back to back classes with no "set up" time in between. In addition, very often classes have been "doubled up" to accommodate the "common planning time concept", and although adequate staffing is sometimes provided, an inordinate demand is being made on the limited facilities, very often, just a multi purpose gym/cafeteria/auditorium facility.

The emphasis on student measurement of learning objectives, which has taken the educational system in this country by storm, has also rushed many physical educators to slap together a written test that measures the cognitive retention of the students.   This has created a patchwork approach to these testing programs.

With this publication, we have made an attempt to help both new and experienced teachers deal with these ever present challenges. We have documented a plethora of activities with the basic physical skills (movement, throwing, catching and/or kicking) as the universal theme, and also provides for increased repetitions for students during each session (i.e. no more waiting on long lines) which we know inhibits skill development.. It is our recommendation that knowledge of these skills can consistently be used to evaluate student learning cognitively (via a written test). Many of the physical education tests that we have examined test <u>game rules</u> and general <u>health education material</u> (bones of the body, systems, etc.) . While some of this material is helpful to know, is it really what you are teaching, or does it belong in the "health curriculum?"

We have included scores of activities appropriate for the never ending addition of students requiring Physical Education who are coming into our schools prior to kindergarten. We have also taken the best activities and their modifications from **Jim's** extensive library, one that he has developed over the 40+ years that he has spent in the profession, and provide the reader with a **"user friendly"** "problem solving" publication that will be an invaluable tool to both experienced and novice physical educators.

The activities presented have been **tried and tested** in less than perfect conditions, are easy to implement, and most importantly: THE KIDS LOVE THEM! We have broken down and listed the basic components of the physical skills that we believe should be learned by all Physical Education students. Feel free to incorporate these components into any written tests that you are asked to develop. Of course, this is by no means a complete list of the skills your students will develop through your curriculum, but they do provide a sound beginning basis for cognitive measurement. Have fun, we assure you that your students will!

Best Regards,

Tom & Jim

Dedication

We would like to dedicate this book to our wives, Dianne and Janet, who encouraged and supported us throughout this project. Also, to the literally tens of thousands of students who we have had the honor of teaching and coaching, and to thank them for allowing us to be part of their lives. Finally, to the teachers and coaches who took a special interest in us during our early years and demonstrated to us, the tremendous influence they can have in shaping their student's future.

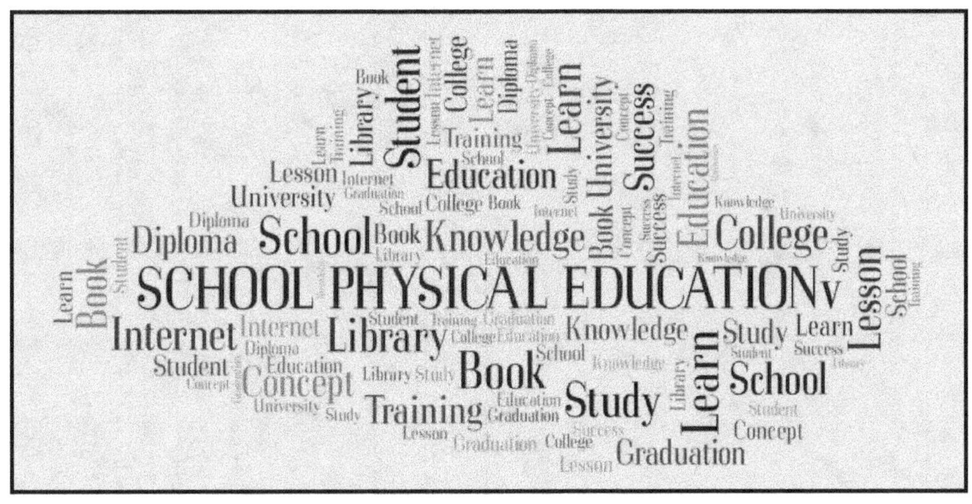

Table Of Contents

Movement Games

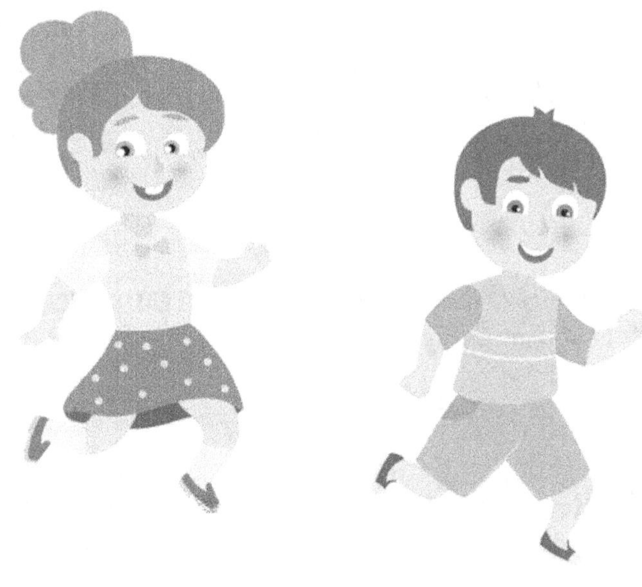

Movement Games

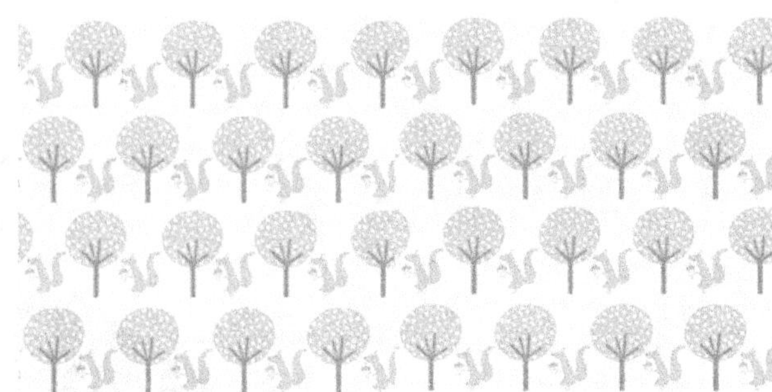

" *Squirrels In The Trees* "

Grade Level: K-2

Equipment: None

Formation: Scatter

How to Play:

Divide the class into groups of threes. Groups numbers 1 & 2 join hands to represent hollow trees, and number 3 stand between them representing squirrels. There should be at least one Squirrel without a home. On a signal from the teacher, all Squirrels must change "trees". The homeless Squirrel attempts to get a tree during the change. After a short period of time change numbers and places.

Outcomes:
Improved Leg Strength, Agility Improvement, Spatial Awareness

Modifications
Because so many kids are inactive playing this game the traditional way, here is a recommendation to improve it. Every student stands in a hoop (each hoop represents a tree). To start, no one gets caught. Because there is one hoop (tree) for every student. When the teacher yells "Squirrel's change trees", everyone leaves their "tree" and finds a new one. Once they get the hang of it, eliminate one tree. The person without a hoop, stands in the middle of the gym. Now on the signal, only one gets caught each round, and everyone is moving. Also, to build upon this game and make it more interesting and fun, play the game:

"Squirrels In A Tree" (Gathering Nuts)

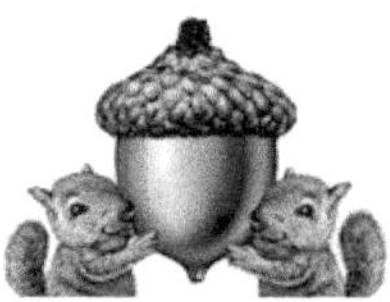

How to Play:

Divide the hoops up into three different colors (Red, Yellow, Blue). Have 3 different color balls (Red, Yellow, Blue). Throw all the balls out onto the playing area, and on the teacher's signal, the students are allowed to pick up any colored ball and return it to the tree of the same color. Start the game with enough trees and nuts for every student. Once the students get the idea of matching the nuts to the corresponding trees, the teacher eliminates one red, one yellow, and one blue hoop (tree). Now, all students still find a nut, but three of them each round are always "caught" without a tree. To start each round, have all of the Squirrels throw the ball somewhere around the gym. The teacher should give two commands: "throw" and then "go" to control class movement in a safe manner.

"Bonus Ball" Movement Games

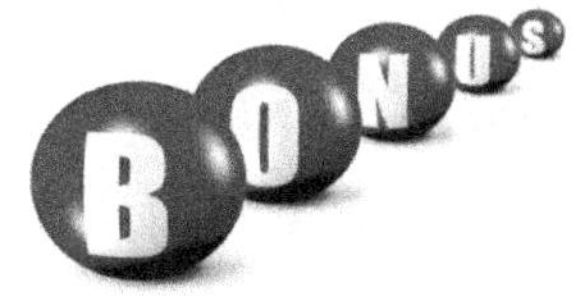

Grade Level: K-6

Equipment: 1 tennis ball for each team plus one extra ball (Mark with marking pen: 1, 2, 3, 4, X)

Formation: Four teams filed behind a line

Outcomes: Improved Leg Strength, Agility Improvement, Directionality, Number Recognition, Propulsion.

How to Play:

The first person in line is given a tennis ball with the team number on it which he/she shows to their teammates. The ball with the "X" , the "bonus ball" is also shown by the teacher. The teacher now collects all of the tennis balls and throws them to the other end of the gym. On the signal from the teacher, the first player in each line runs to retrieve his team's ball. Once the player has found the numbered ball belonging to his team, he returns it to the next player in line (Carried back, not thrown). If, in the process of looking for their ball, they happen to pick up a ball belonging to another team, they will throw it off the side wall of the gym. This would be done to slow down another team in the competition. After returning their team's ball, the player starts out again in search of the **"bonus ball"**. Once it is in their possession, they raise the **"bonus ball"** over their head , and then the teacher blows the whistle and that player wins the round. Play then proceeds with the next players in line taking their turn.

<u>Modifications:</u>

*A great lead up game to this is a game we named **"<u>One Less</u>"**.   If there are 6 teams, the instructor takes (5) unmarked tennis balls and throws them to the other end of the gym. On a signal from the instructor (usually given when the balls are in motion) all 5 students run out and pick up <u>any</u> ball and raise it in the air (no need to run it back). Everyone gets a ball except one. Then bring back the balls to the instructor, and go to the end of the line. **<u>A second variation</u>** is also fun...Six players (can be played with any number) line up behind six "marked" cones. This variation is called :*

"Random Numbered Ball"

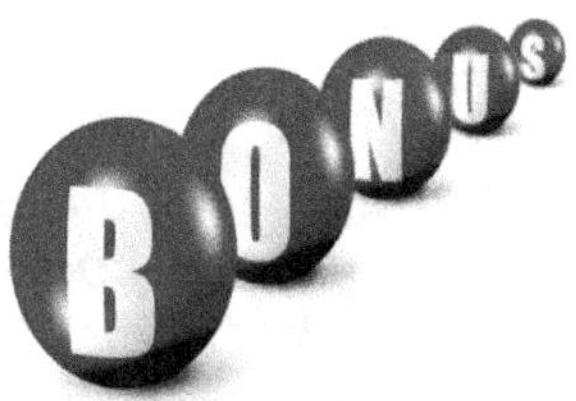

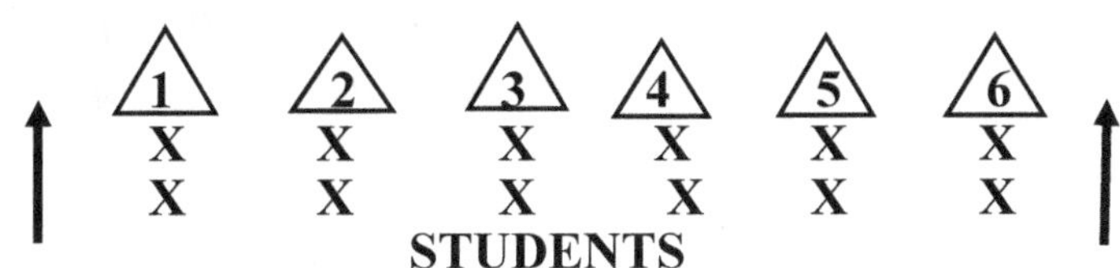

Continued……..

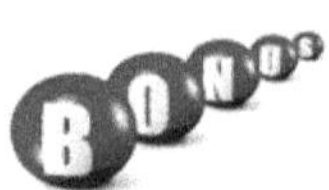

Movement Games

"Bonus Ball "
Continued.....

*The instructor throws out balls marked 1 thru 6. All 6 students run out and pick up the first ball they come upon, look at the number on the ball, and run it back to the cone that is marked with the same number. This now becomes their new team for their next chance. Chances are students will pick up a number other than their original team on each opportunity. **Note:** this is a great game for number recognition with the early childhood students. Playing all three of these games (One Less, Random Numbered Ball, Bonus Ball) during the same period will provide the instructor with an excellent lesson.*

"Forest Lookout"

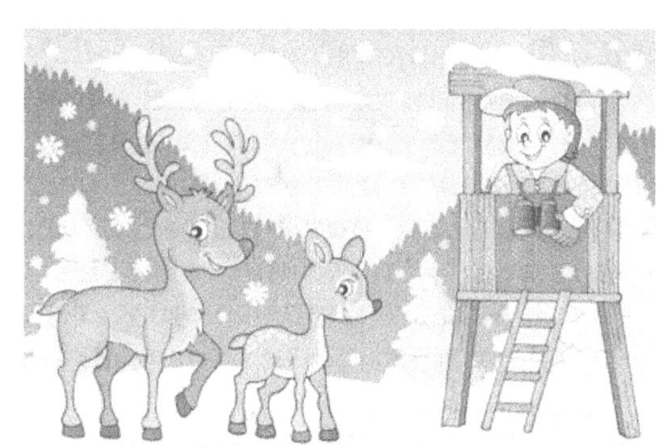

Grade Level: K-2

Equipment: 1 less hoop than # of students

Formation: Circle

How to Play:

The hoops are placed around the perimeter of the gym and represent trees. The students each line up behind a tree. The **"forest ranger"** takes his place in the center and says, "Fire in the mountains—"run, run, run" or ("walk," "hop," "jump," "skip," "gallop." or "slide") and joins the rest of the group as they move around the gym clockwise behind the trees (hoops). When they have gone around the gym once or twice, the teacher blows the whistle indicating **"the fire is out**," and everyone tries to find a tree. All students can run in any direction to find a tree after the whistle (there is always one less tree than the number of students). For the next round the teacher will pick someone who has successfully found an open tree to be the next forest ranger.

Modifications:
*I have found that playing this traditional game in a large square area makes much better use of your space, and students get an increased amount of movement. The teacher always picks the next **"forest ranger"** from someone who successfully found a tree in order to increase student motivation. This variation makes this a "Super Fun Game" for early childhood (grades K-2).*

"Whistle Mixer"

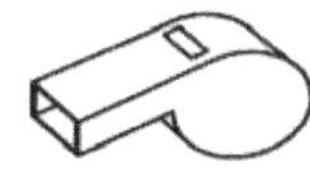

Movement Games

Grade Level: 1-3

Equipment: Whistle, Tom-Tom

Formation: Students are scattered throughout area.

Outcomes: Improved Leg Strength, Agility Improvement, balance, directionality.

How to Play:

To begin, students walk around in any direction they wish. The teacher blows a whistle a number of tines in succession with short, sharp blasts. Whatever the number of blasts, the children form small circles with the number in the circle equal to the number established by the whistle signal. Thus, if there are four blasts, the children form circles of four—no more, no less.

Any children left out are eliminated. Also, if a circle is formed with more than the specified number, the entire circle is eliminated. After the circles have been formed and the eliminated children have been moved to the sidelines, the teacher calls, "Walk" and the game continues. In walking, the children should move in different directions.

<u>Modification</u>

This game is a good warm up activity, but should not be used as an entire lesson. An advanced version of this game can be done with the aid of a tom-tom different beats of the tom-tom would indicate various locomotor movements i.e. skipping, galloping, slow walk, normal walk, running. The whistle would still be used to set the number to be in each circ

"Touchdown"

Grade Level: 1-6

Equipment: One object small enough to conceal in one hand (a coin works well)

Outcomes: Agility, Balance

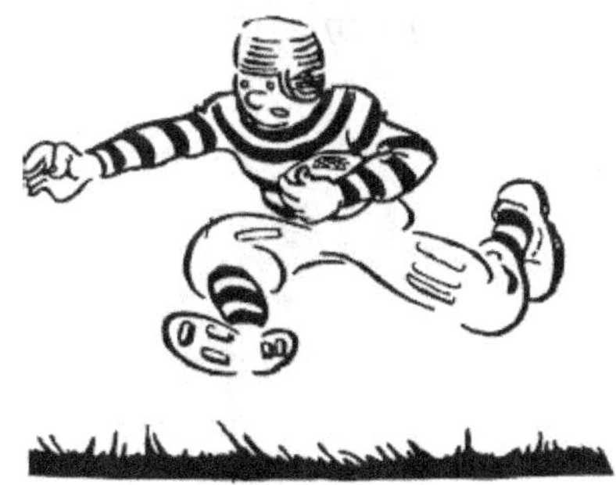

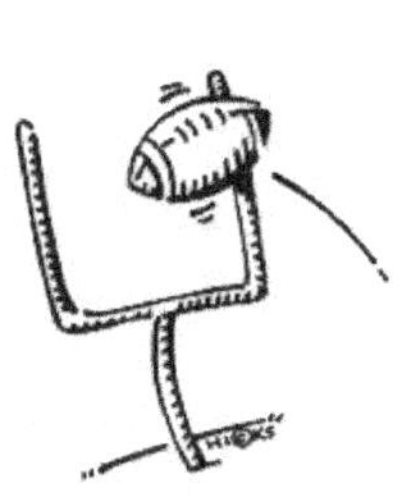

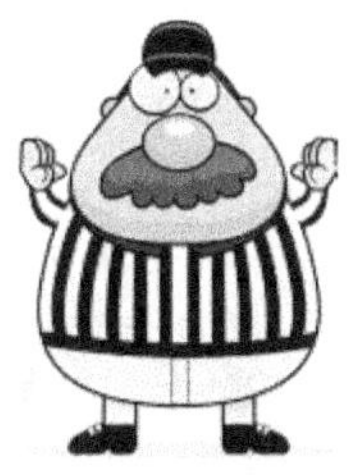

Continued........

"Touchdown "

Continued...

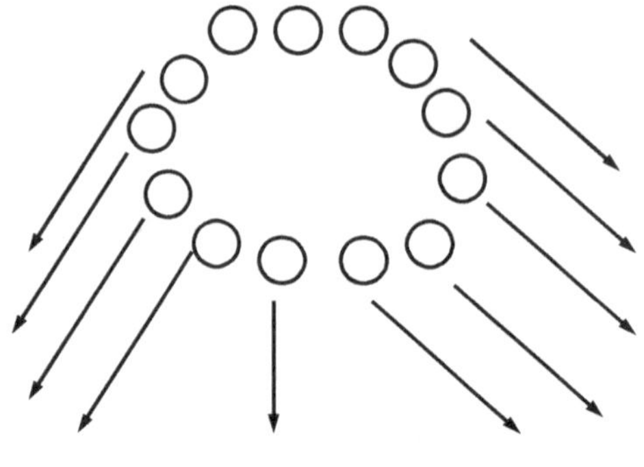

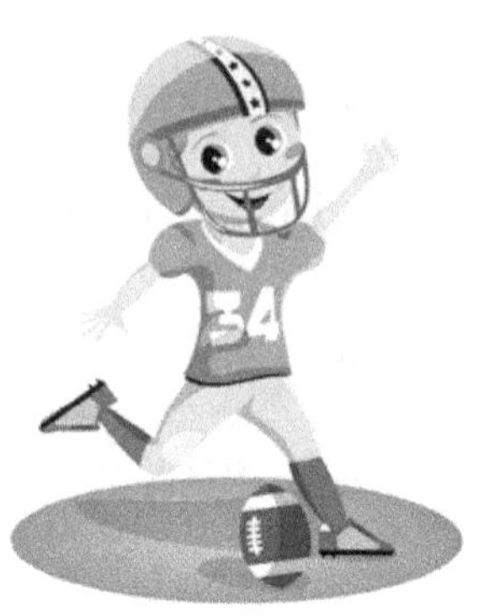

How to Play:

The game begins with a flip of the coin to decide which team has first possession of the "ball' (coin). Each team goes to its own goal line. The team with the ball goes into a huddle and their opponents space themselves as shown. The team in the huddle gives the ball to one player who closes both hands, concealing it in one. All players on that team pretend to have the ball by closing both hands. The object of the game is to carry the ball across the opponents goal line without being tagged. As soon as the team with the ball comes out of its huddle to attempt to score, the opposing team advances toward them and tries to tag as many of them as possible. Each person tagged must stop and show both opened hands to the one who tagged him before either can rejoin the game.

If the player with the ball is tagged, the next game continues with the opposing team in possession of the ball. If, however, the player with the ball crosses the opponents' goal line without being tagged, he scores a touchdown, earning six points for his team. The game continues as in the beginning with the teams taking turns at attempting to score.

Modifications

Although this game is intended for early childhood students, it has also been very successful with grades 4-6. It is especially fun around "Super Bowl" time where the class can be broken up and given the names of the two super bowl opponents.

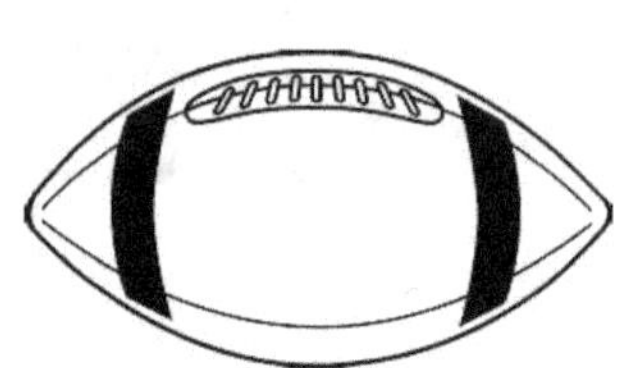

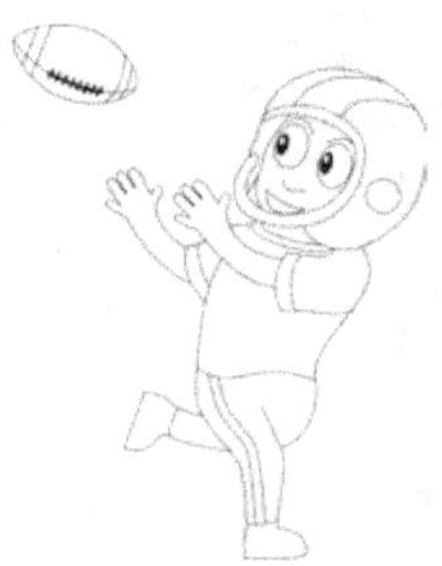

Movement Games

"Steal The Bacon"

Grade Level: K-6 (This game is geared for the younger students, but played up to grade 6)

Equipment: 1 bowling pin

Formation: Two lines 20' or more apart: one team behind each line.

Outcomes: Improved Leg Strength, Agility Improvement, Directionality

How to Play:

The bowling pin is set in a circle in the center. The players count off so that each player has a number. The instructor calls a number. The player having that number from each team runs out. Each attempts to snatch the bowling pin and return to his position in line before the other can tag him. The player may make several false moves to get his opponent off balance before he succeeds in snatching the pin. The pin is replaced and another number is called. Two points are awarded to the team whose player succeeds in snatching the pin and returning to his line without being tagged. One point is awarded to the player that tags the other before he returns to his line with the pin. The team with the highest score at the conclusion of the game wins...

<u>**Modifications:**</u>
I play this game mostly with Grades K-2 but older grades always find it fun. In order to get more kids involved at one time, I break the playing area down into three (3) separate playing areas as depicted below. When one number is called out, six (6) Players come out (2A's, 2B's and 2C's). As a result three different games are being played at one time. The allows for more kids to participate. After a few rounds, rotate teams so each team can face different opponents during a class period.

A's	B's	C's
◇	◇	◇
A 's	B's	C's

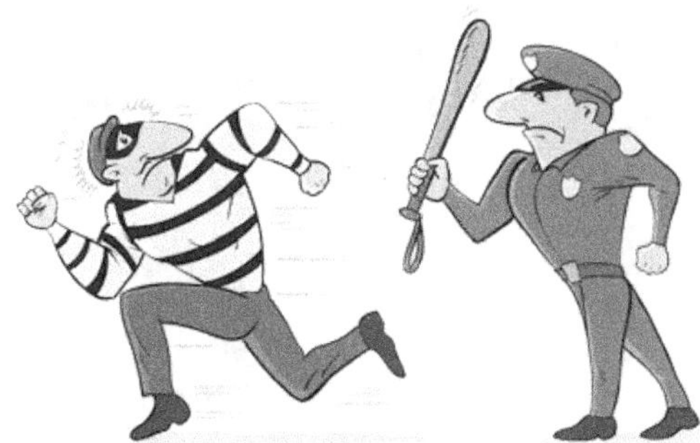

Movement Games

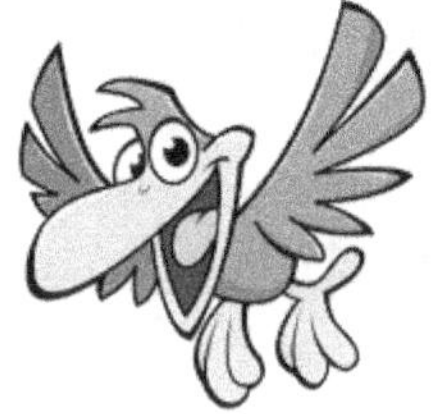

"Bird Catcher"

Grade Level: K-2

Equipment: None

Formation: Circle and line

How to Play:

Half of the class-the "Birds"- line up on a line; the others form a circle (the Nest). Choose one player to be the "Bird Catcher" and station them between the Birds and the Nest. On a signal, the Birds try to get to the Nest before the Catcher tags them. All those tagged become "Bird Catchers". A second signal is then given so that those who have reached the Nest may return to the line without being tagged. The game continues until all are caught. The Nest and Birds change places and the game is replayed

Modifications:

This game can get confusing to young children. For that reason, I have the original "Bird Catcher" wear a colored scrimmage vest. When a bird is tagged, and becomes a bird catcher, he/she also puts on a vest. This makes it easier to distinguish the "birds" from the "catcher"

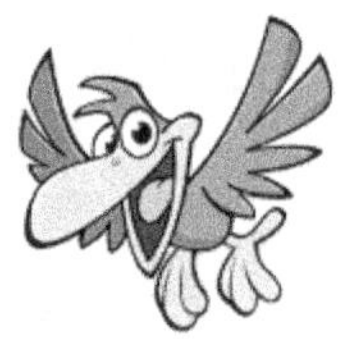

"Coconut Tree"

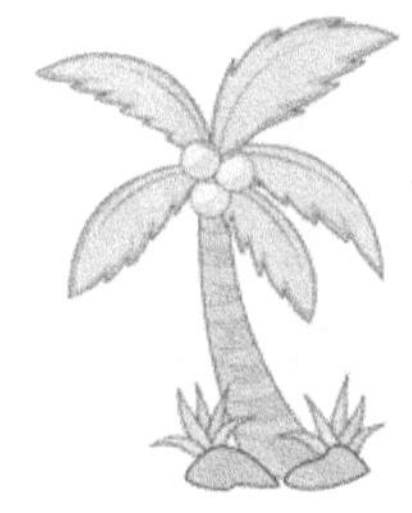

Grade Level: PK-2

Equipment: Hoops (1 per student), Bean Bags (1 per student)

Formation: Each student stand In a hoop with a bean bag

How to Play:

The object of the game is to collect as many beanbags as you can and bring them back to *Your* tree before the whistle blows. A good amount of time is anywhere between 30 seconds and 1 minute (longer than 1 minute will tire the students out to quickly).
The only rules are as follows:

* You may only collect 1 beanbag at a time.

* Freeze on the whistle

* If you have a bean bag in your hand when the whistle blows—you may bring it back to your tree. If not, go back to your tree without one.

When all of the students are back, ask "How many have no coconuts?"
For those raising their hands, explain that it is ok, they will get some the next round.

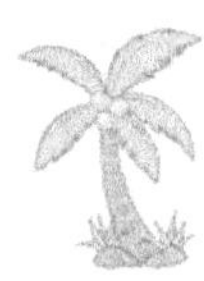

Continued…...

Movement Games

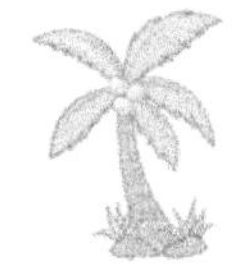

"Coconut Tree" continued....

Modifications:
Because the children get tired quickly, split the group into two even units (birthday months, even/odd, etc.) While one group collects coconuts, the other can rest.

If you are fortunate enough to have colored hoops and beanbags, this is a great way to play:
6 red hoops and beanbags
6 yellow hoops and beanbags
6 yellow hoops and beanbags

Other ways to play:
You can only get the same color coconuts as your hoop.

"Mickey Mouse"

Grade Level: K-2
Equipment: 4 Bowling Pins

Formation: 4 Teams—Each team occupying 1/4 of a half court area. Each player is given a number, and they are seated. 1 bowling pin is stationed in front of each team (the pin in front of the team is the one they have to knock down).

How to Play:
This is a great game for young children to distinguish right from left. Before the game is started, call "left" or "right" and have everyone point in that direction. Check and make any corrections necessary. Once you are satisfied that they all know the difference, begin to explain the game.

Coconut Tree Diagram
X-Student   B– Bean Bag

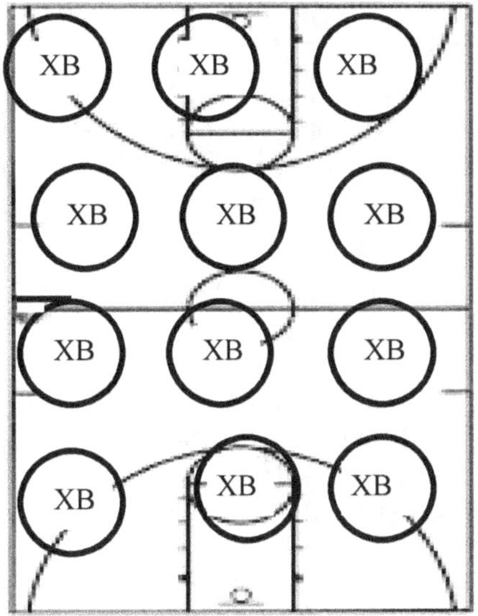

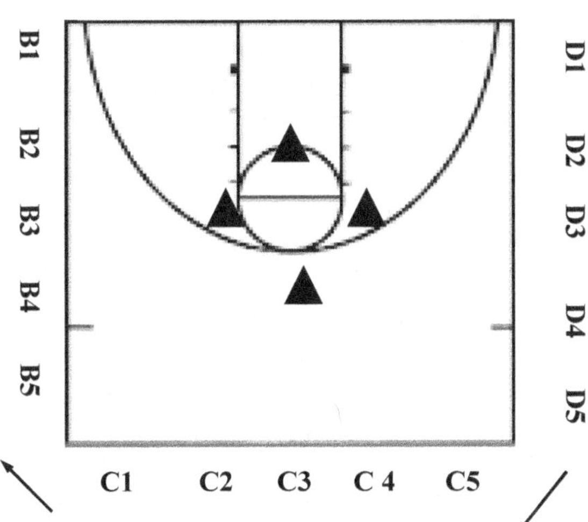

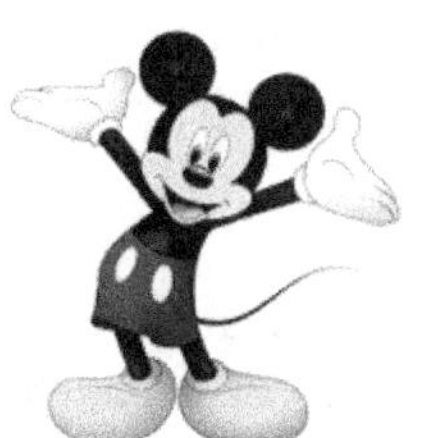

Continued on next page

Movement Games

"Mickey Mouse" 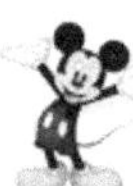 *continued...*

The instructor calls out a direction, and waits 1 second or so to give everyone a chance to know which is which. Then the instructor calls out a number 1 thru 5. Everyone with that number stands up and starts to run around all four teams (explain to students that they must run in a clockwise direction, and demonstrate what "clockwise" means). When they return to their original spot, they run forward to the pin and tip it over (no kicking).

The three teams to tip over a pin first receives the letter "M". The instructor then calls a different number, and the students repeat the same procedure. Giving the three teams who finish first in each round another letter. Play continues until one of the teams receive all the letters in "MICKEY MOUSE"

"Man From Mars"

A - "Man From Mars"

B– Other Class Members (Red, White, Blue)

Grade Level: K-2
Equipment: None
Formation: 1 player who is the "Man From Mars" stands at the opposite foul line from the rest of the class. All other students line up behind the opposite end line, and are given a color (Red, White, Blue).

How to Play:
Facing the entire class the *Man From Mars* chants "I am the Man From Mars, and I will take you to the stars if your color is:
"The player calls out either red, yellow, or blue."

Only those players of that color attempt to cross to the other end line without being tagged by the MFM. Those who are tagged will stop and raise their hand. Upon completion of each run, all those who were tagged will join those who made it safely, and a second color is called. After the MFM has had 3 tries, choose a new one.

Tip: Use colored vests if you have them (Young children sometimes forget their color. Safety: No running outside the sidelines.

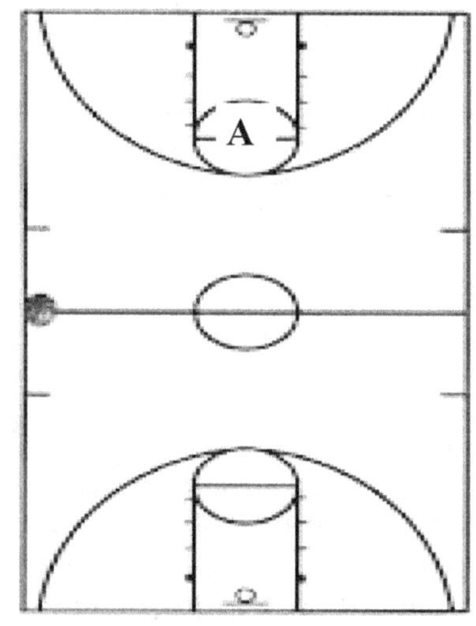

BBBBBBBBBBBBBBBB

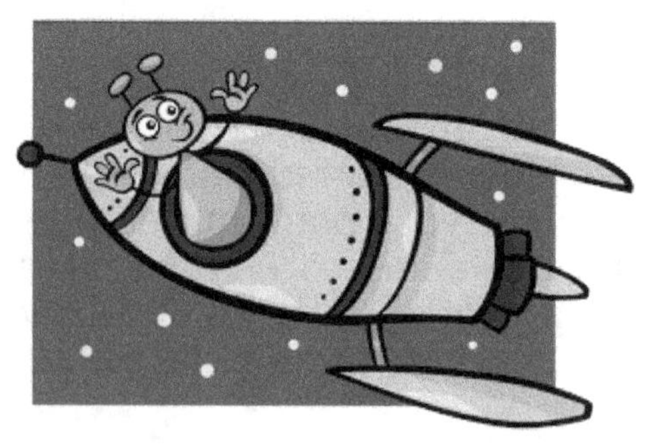

Movement Games

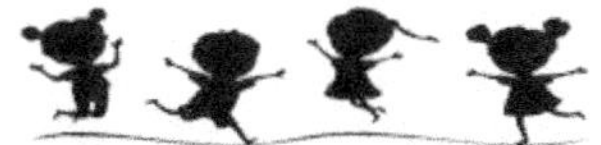

"Hoop Color Tag"

Grade Level: K-2

Equipment: 1 Hoop for each student. (3 different color hoops).

Formation: Hoops are scattered around the gym, each student standing in one. One person is the "tagger" who stands in the center of the gym.

How to Play:

When the instructor calls out a color "tagger" attempts to tag as many players as they can before they find another hoop. When tagged, they must stop and raise their hand. Upon completion, those tagged may find a hoop, and the next color is called. After the tagger has had 3 turns, choose another "Tagger".

"Ghostbuster Tag"

Grade Level: K-2

Equipment: None

Formation: Only half the court is used (no one is allowed out the lines) One person is designated as the 'tagger" who stands on the foul line. All other students scatter away from the "tagger" staying within the boundary lines.

How to Play:

This is a great warm up activity that can be played for a few minutes before your main activity. On the signal "go" the tagger attempts to tag as many as they can in a certain time frame (30 seconds works well). When tagged you must go to the "tagged area" and sit. Continue until the whistle blows, then choose a new tagger. Students are only allowed to <u>walk.</u> Tagger can wear a vest to identify them. Also, you can add more taggers.

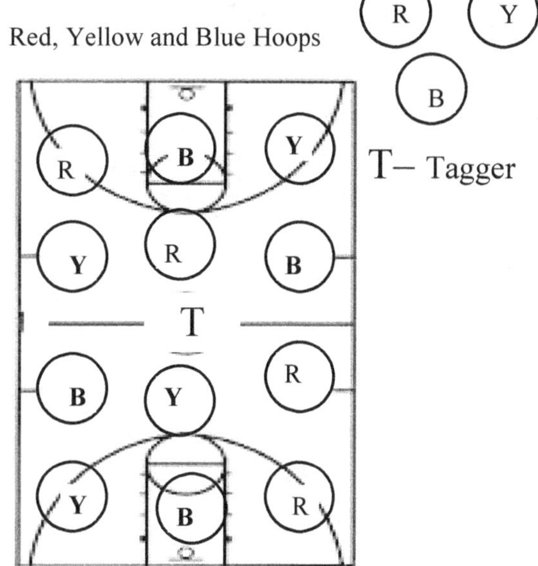
Red, Yellow and Blue Hoops

"Hoop Color Tag Diagram

TIP: After awhile you may want to add two colors on each call, and for more of a challenge add all three.

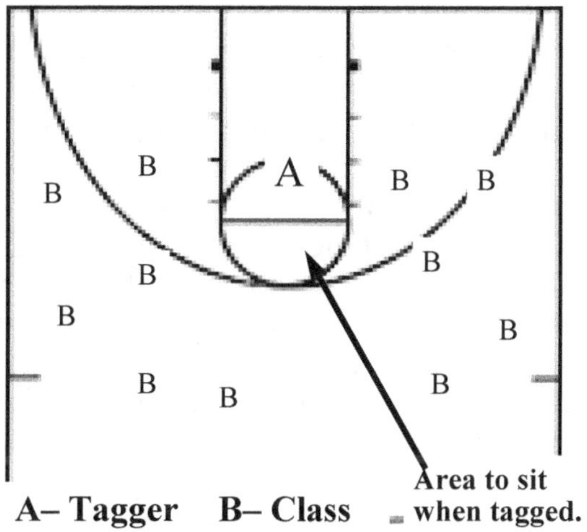

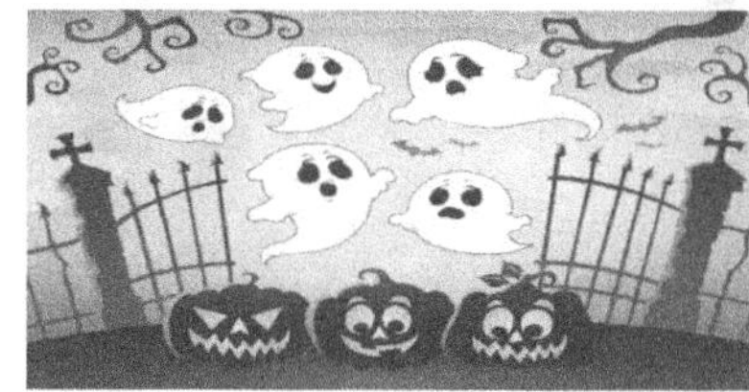

"Bean Bag Change"

Grade Level: K-2
Equipment: 2 Bean Bags
Formation: Two lines 40' apart, one team behind each line.

1 2 3 4 5 6 7 8 9

O   O   O   40 Feet

9 8 7 6 5 4 3 2 1

How to Play:

Two equal teams are consecutively numbered beginning from opposite ends of each line. Mark three one foot circles midway between the two teams, one at the center and the other two at the ends. The center circle is common to both teams, but the teacher assigns one of the end circles to each team.

Place two beanbags in the center circle. The teacher then calls out a number. The individual from each team having that number runs to the center circle. Each picks up one beanbag, transfers it to his team's assigned circle, and returns to his original position. The runner returning first scores a point for their team. The next number is called and the new runners transfer the beanbags back to the center circle. The runner returning first scores one point for their team. The game is complete when all numbers have been called.

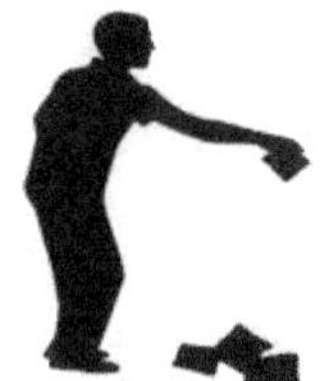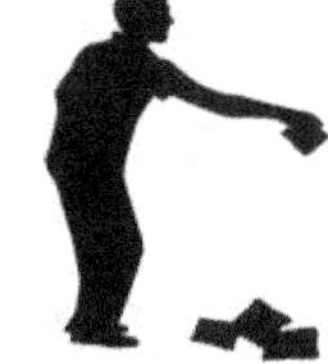

Movement Games

'Double Bean Bag Change"

Equipment: 4 Bean Bags
Formation: Two lines 40' apart, one team behind each line

1 2 3 4 5 6 7 8 9

O
O   O   O   40 Feet
O

9 8 7 6 5 4 3 2 1

How to Play:

Two equal teams are consecutively numbered beginning from opposite ends of each line. Mark 5 one foot circles, placing three circles midway and perpendicular to the lines of the players, the two other circles midway between the teams and three feet outside the ends of the lines. The center circle is common to both teams, but the other circles are assigned by the teacher.

Place four beanbags in the center circle. The teacher calls a number. Both individuals having that number run to the center circle. Each picks up one beanbag and transfers it to their team's circle on the end, then returns to the center circle for his second beanbag and places it in the circle in front of his team. The first runner to return to his starting position scores a point for his team. When the next number is called, the new runners transfer the beanbags back to the center circle.

Tip: This game works great as a relay also. After it is played the regular way, try it as a relay....

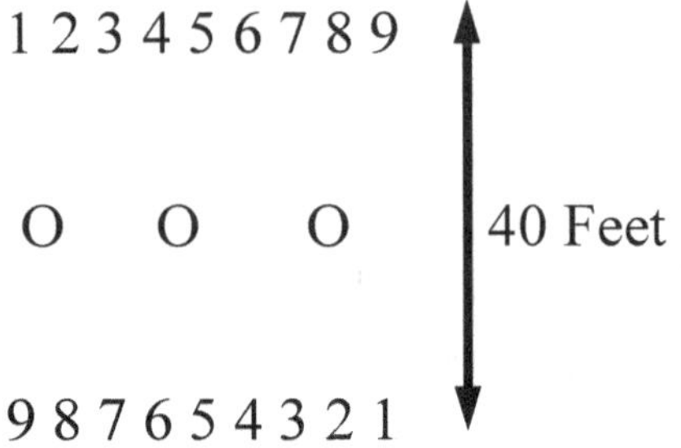
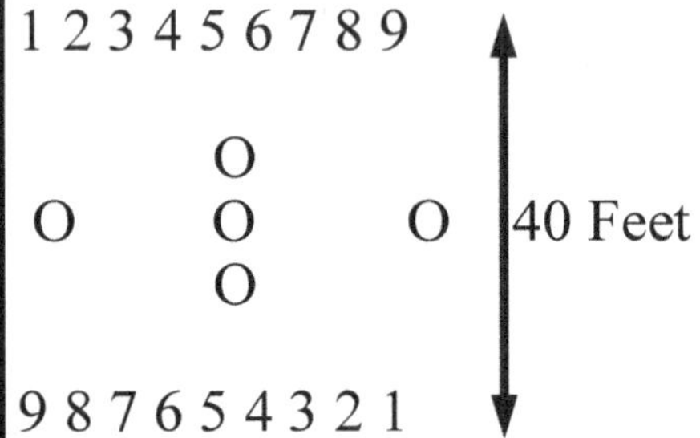

Movement Games

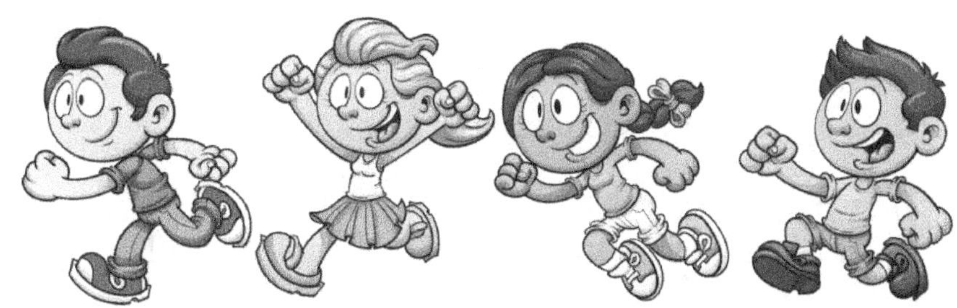

"Water Sprite"

Grade Level: K-2

Equipment: None

Formation: 4 equal teams, each occupying 1/4 of the 1/2 court.

How to Play:
This is a very simple game that can be used effectively as a "warm up." The instructor calls out any number 1 thru 5. Everyone with that number attempts to get across to the other side without getting tagged. Anyone getting tagged, must stop and raise their hand. Change taggers so everyone gets a turn.

Tip: Numbered poly-spots are great for this game so the runners are told to run to the poly spot that is empty.

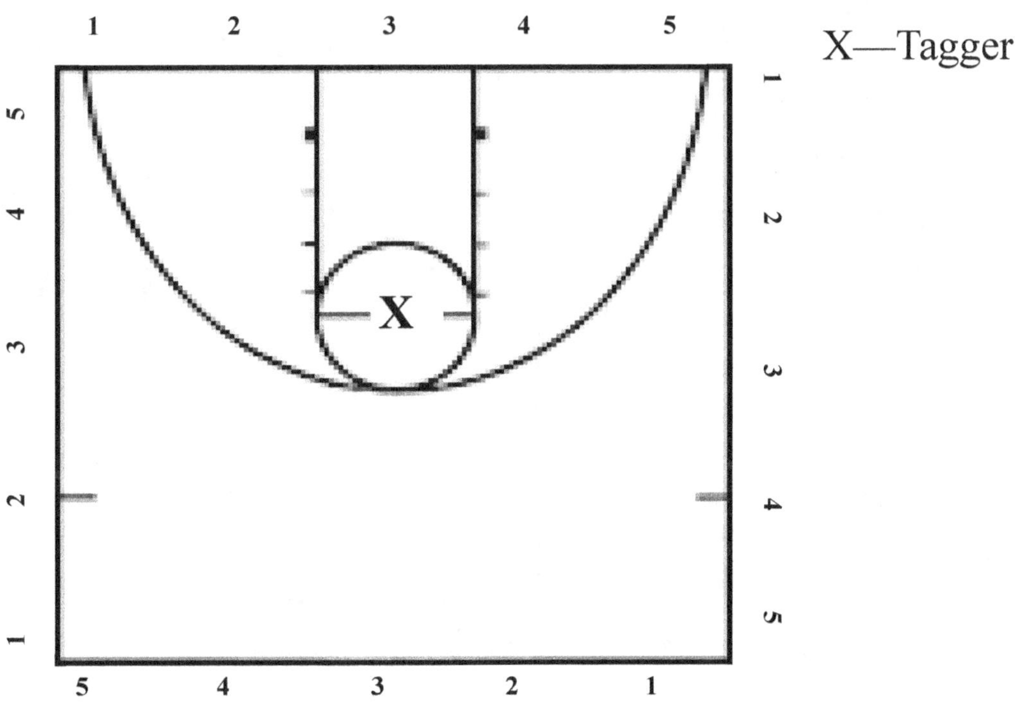

"Club Snatch" Movement Games

Grade Level: K-2
Equipment: 3 Clubs or Bowling Pins

Formation: The gym is divided into 3 areas (see diagram). Each area has 2 teams facing each other with an assigned number. A club or bowling pin is placed closer to one side than the other.

How to Play:

This is a good lead-up game to "steal the bacon" When a number is called, the team member closer to the pin runs out and attempts to pick up the pin and get back to the goal line without being tagged by the opposing team. After 3 rounds, switch the pin or club so that it is closer to the other side and continue.

Tip: I like to rotate teams after a while so that everyone gets a chance to go against different opponents.

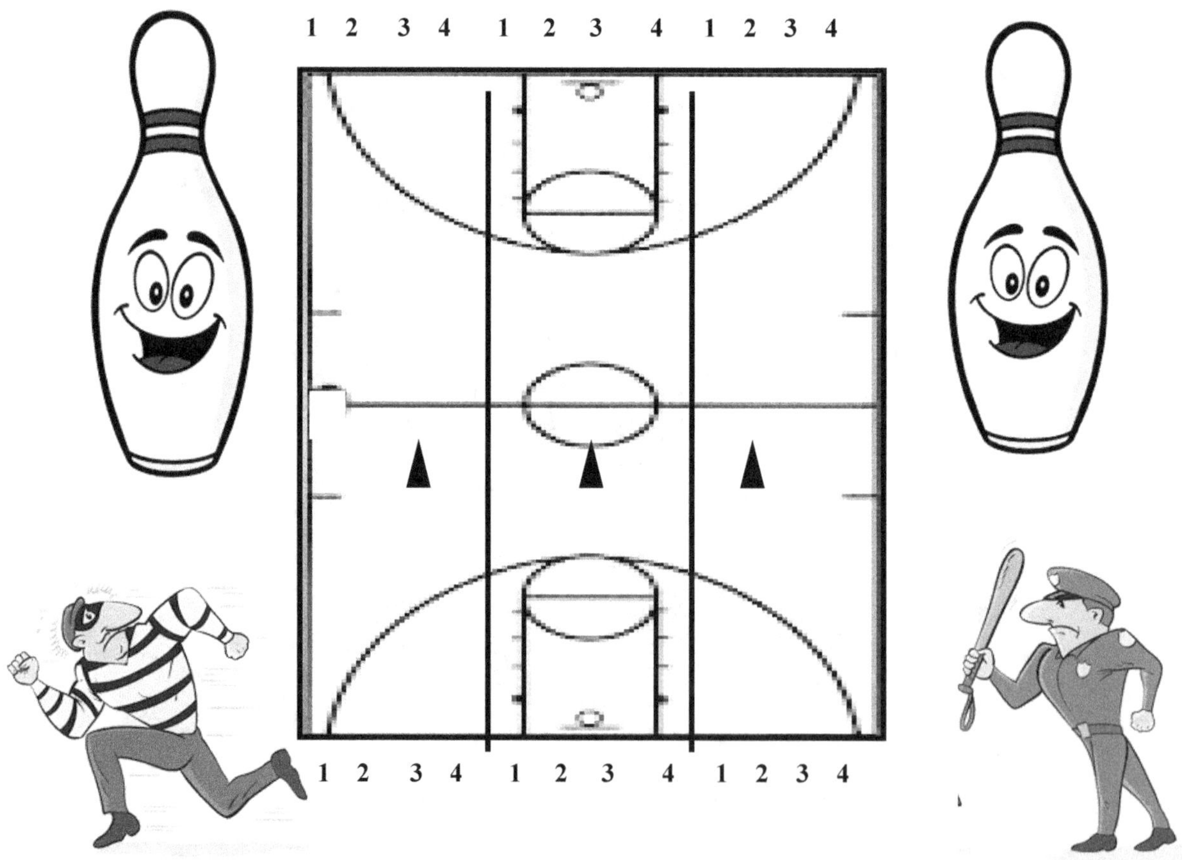

Kicking Games

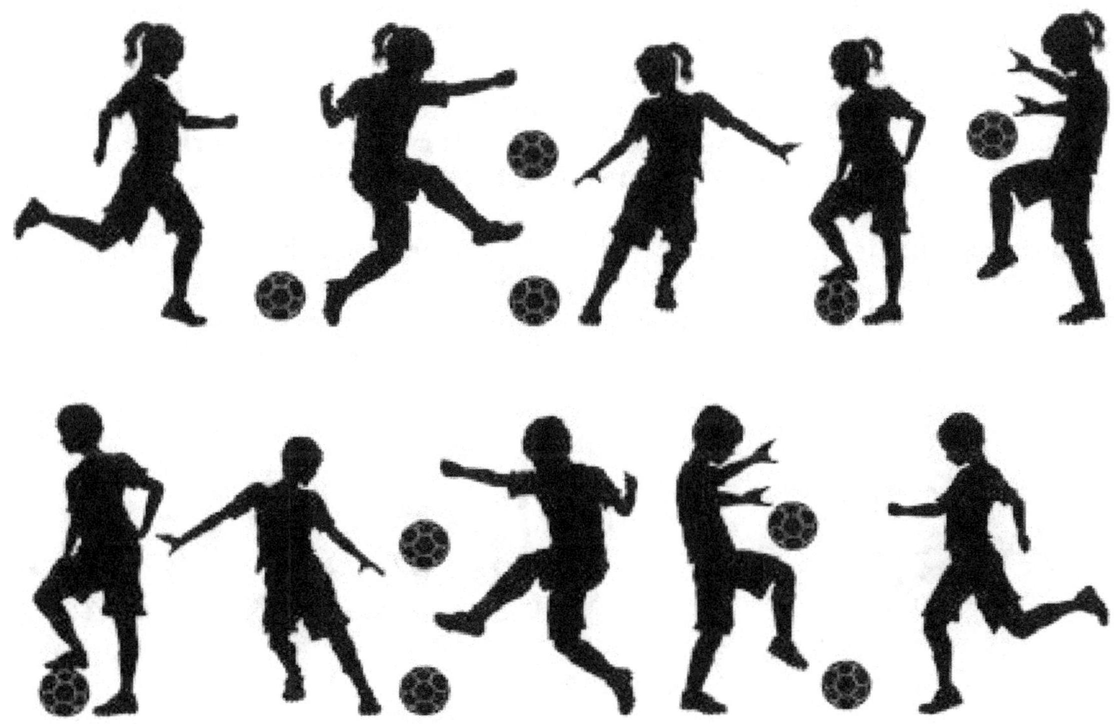

Kicking Games

"Red - Yellow - Blue Kickball"

Equipment: 3 balls of the <u>same</u> color (each marked with a different number (1, 2, or 3), 3 Cones, at half court, and 3 bases.

For those of you looking for a great Kicking game, look no further! "Red, Yellow, Blue Kickball", "1,2,3, Kickball", and "Mystery Kickball" are progressive games from "easy" (K-1) to "challenging" (3-Up).

How to Play:

Three "kickers" kick at the same time on the signal "go". Once all the balls have been kicked, the "kickers" run straight to the "half-court" line, run around the cone directly in front of them, and back to the "kicking line" (Not to the base...this is explained below). Whoever catches the ball must throw it to the correct base. Red ball to the catcher by the red base, yellow to yellow, blue to blue. If the kicker crosses the "kicking line" before the catcher receives the ball and steps on the appropriate base they are safe, if not they are out. **Note: The reason the kicker does not run to the base is to avoid collisions.**

After all three have kicked, the rotation is as follows: 1. **All 3 kickers go to the end of the line and the next three kickers who are waiting are called** (They are all given numbers before the game starts). The "catchers" and "fielders" rotate as follows: 1 follows 2, 2 follows 3, etc. 9 will replace 1. **Play continues until all the fielders are back at their original positions. At this time kickers become fielders and vice versa.**

Modifications: Explain to the "kickers" that the further they kick the ball the better chance theY have of scoring safely. Let the fielders know that if the ball is kicked deep, they may want to relay it in to a teammate. Once your class plays this game, introduce:

"Kickball 123" (SEE NEXT PAGE)

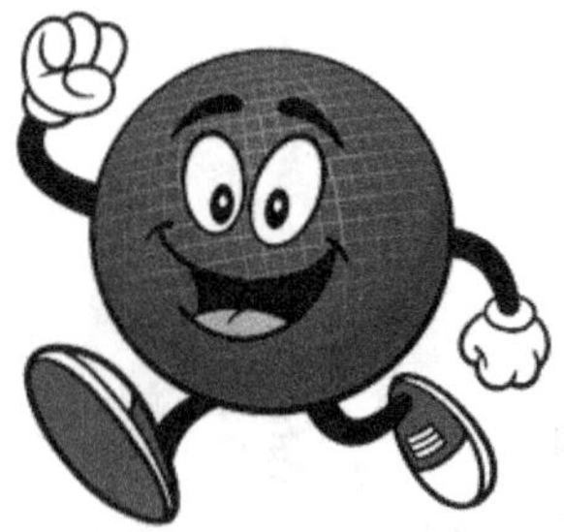

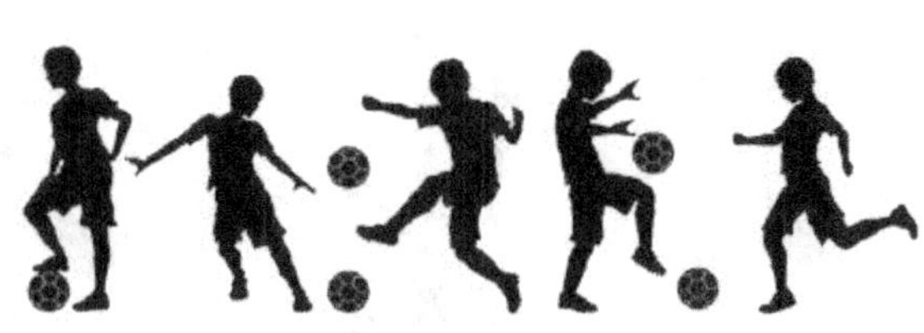

"Kickball 1, 2, 3 "   Kicking Games

Grades K-5
Formation: One Kicker lined up behind each ball.
The rest of the fielding team spread out starting at the half court line in 3 rows.
Equipment: 3 balls of the <u>same</u> color (each marked with a different number (1, 2, or 3), 3 Cones at half court, and 3 bases. **(See diagram on previous page)**

How to Play:
Everything is the same as "R,Y,B Kickball" except the first kicker has to kick #1, the middle kicker has to kick #2, and the last kicker has to kick #3. Since all the balls are the same color, the fielders now must locate the number on the ball, then throw to the correct base. Scoring and rotating are the same as in "R-Y-B"

Modifications:
Have the fielders "call out" the number to get the "catchers" attention. After class, tell the children "Get ready next time to play one of the best games they will ever play" **MYSTERY KICKBALL!**

"Mystery Kickball " **?????????????????**

Grades 3-6
Formation: Same as Diagram For "R-Y-B Kickball" except **Any Numbered Ball** may be given to any numbered Kicker **(ex. Kicker number one, might be given Ball #2)**
Equipment: (3 Balls Marked #1,#2, #3) , (3 Cones Marked #1,#2, #3,) and 3 bases.

How to Play: Once the kickers are standing behind the kicking line, the teacher will throw each kicker a ball who will place it on the line. The "Kicker" may get any of the three balls (#'s 1,2, or 3). Here's the challenging part: **Whatever ball you kick, you <u>Must</u> *Run Around That Numbered Cone* and back to that "Kicking Line."**

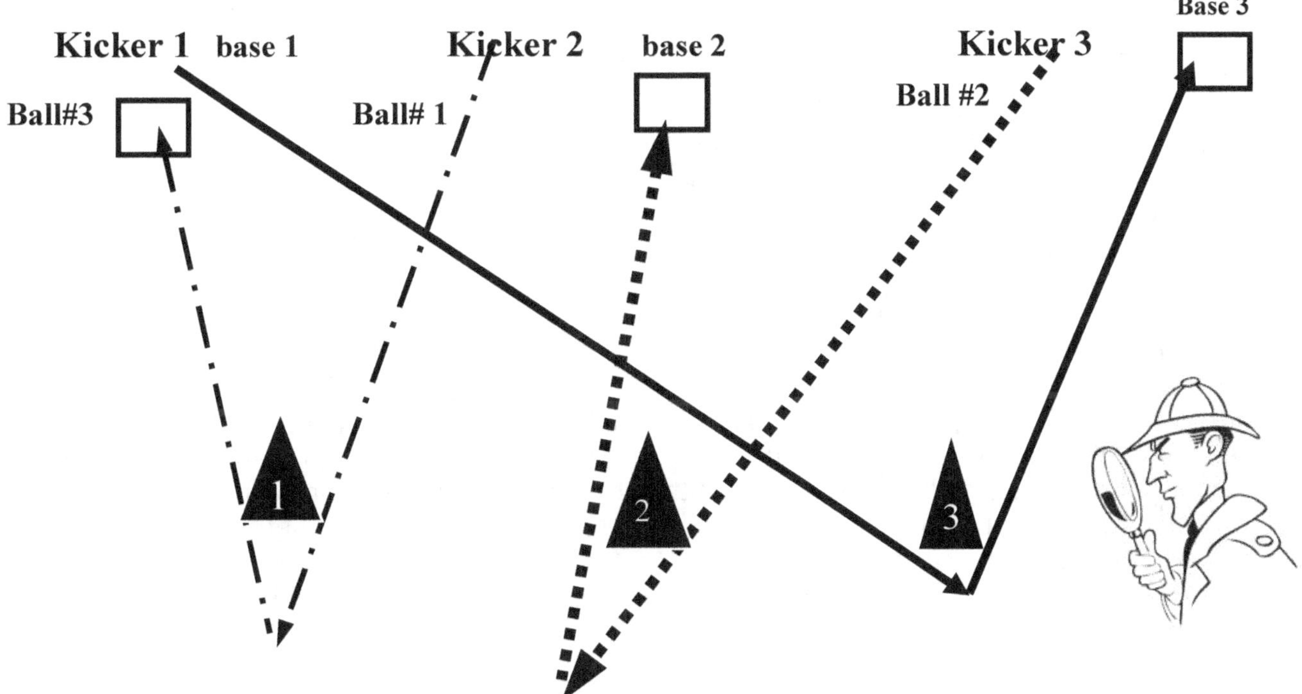

"Mystery Kickball ???" continued....   Kicking Games

TIPS: For whatever reason, the "kickers" want to run back to where they started, no matter what cone they ran around. What I find works is to tell the kicker **"when you circle the correct cone, just run straight back."** I usually play this game for 2 weeks because it does take time to explain, and mistakes are made quite often. However, once the class gets it right, they love it and will want to play it all the time!!

R-Y-B Kickball: Kickers run to the cone directly in front of them and directly back.

1-2-3 Kickball: Kickers again run to the cone directly in front of them and directly back.

Mystery Kickball: Mark cones #1, #2, #3 so kickers can see them.
Explain the **main rule:** "You must run to 2 different places, first the cone with the number of the ball you kick on it, then straight back to the proper kicking line."

"Alaskan Kickball "

Grades 2-5
Formation: See Diagram
Equipment: Kickball, 4 cones,
         1 Home Plate

How to Play:

Depending on the skill level, you may wish to have the ball kicked from a stationary position, or have it rolled by the teacher.

Once the ball is kicked, the kicker starts to run in <u>back</u> of each cone, starting with the **#1 cone**. The kicker will continue to run until the whistle is blown. One point is awarded for every cone that the kicker runs behind.

If **home plate** is passed the kicker can continue to run until the instructor blows the whistle. To stop the kicker from continuing to score: whoever catches the ball, stops at the spot where the catch was made. All of the other fielders must line up in a straight line behind that person as quickly as possible. Once that is done, the person who caught the ball will pass the ball overhead to the person in line behind them. When the last person in line gets the ball, they run to the

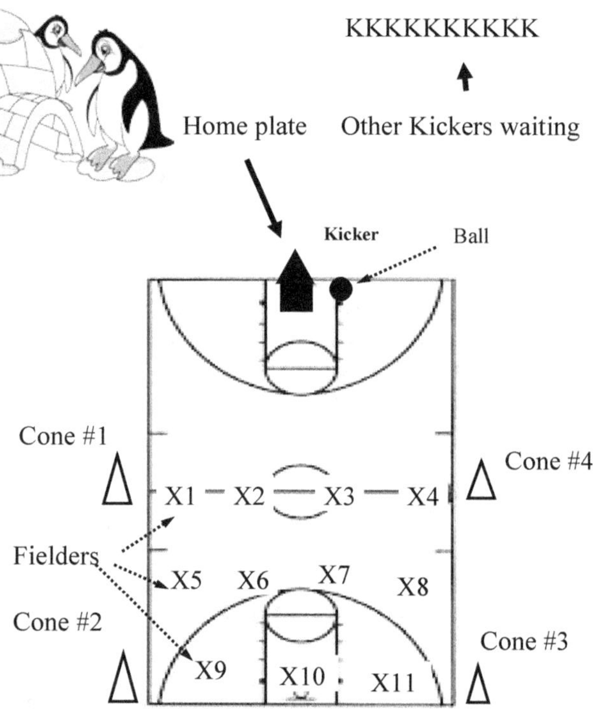

front and stand in front of the first person, signaling the whistle to blow. One point is awarded to the kicking team for each cone passed before the whistle. All members of the kicking team get a chance before the teams switch sides. Fielders rotate to the next spot after each kick.

Continued.........

Alaskan Kickball " Continued.....   **Kicking Games**

TIP: Because the fielders are going to rush to keep the kicker from scoring a lot of points, explain that there will be penalties for the following mistakes:

1. One extra point for handing the ball sideways instead of overhead.

2. One point for everyone who doesn't touch the ball (this occurs when people are slow lining up.

3. This is the WORST!! If the ball should drop to the ground, the person closest to it, will pick it up, run to the front ,and start all over. When this happens, I have seen kickers score 8 to 10 points.

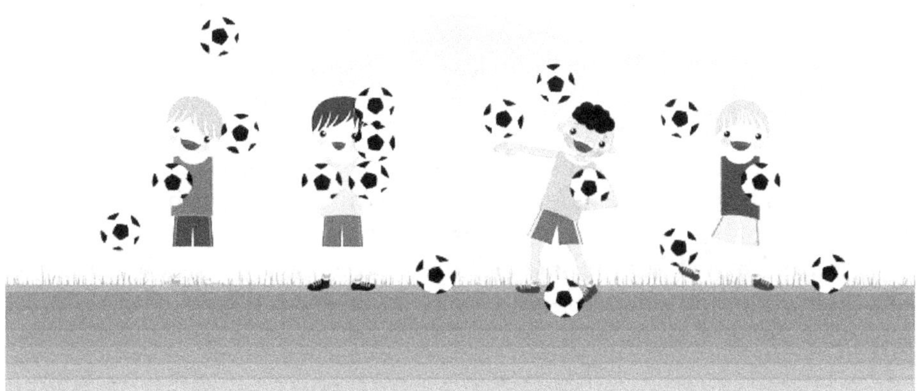

"Line Soccer"

Line Soccer

Grades 3-6

Formation: 2 teams consisting of 3 groups.
1. <u>Scorers</u> on the court, cannot cross sidelines or goal line or beyond it.
2. <u>Goalies</u> cannot step over the goal line.
3. <u>Sideline players</u> cannot step over sideline.

Equipment: 1 Nerf soccer ball.

How to Play:
The scorers attempt to score a goal by kicking the ball over the goal line within a certain hight restriction (6'-8') marked on the wall.

Continued............

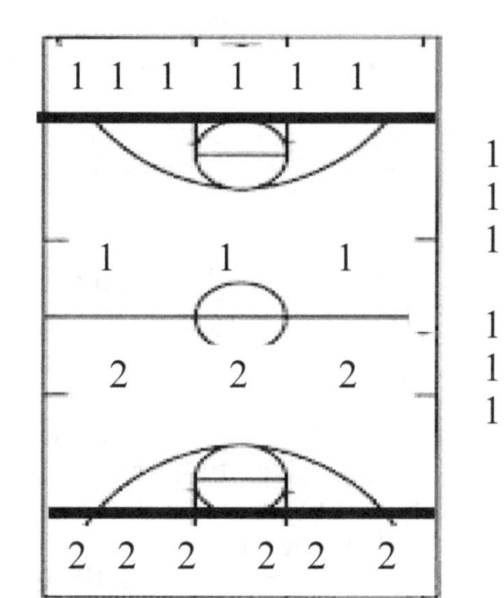

"Line Soccer" continued.....

Any ball kicked over the sideline may be picked up (hands may be used by sideline players) and passed back to one of the scorers. A goalie making a save may pass it back to one of their scorers or directly to a sideline player if the scorers are covered. Any goal scored will result in a point, and the goalie passes it to either a scorer or sideline to continue. (No need to line back up after a goal).
Play continues for 1 minute. Upon completion of the minute rotate the following way:

3 scorers become 3 sideline players ➔ 3 sideline players become last 3 goalies ➔ next 3 goalies in line become scorers.

Tips:
- Adding sideline players gets more people involved creates more scoring opportunities. The only players who cannot use their hands are the scorers.
- A scorer using their hands will result in a penalty. The clock stops and the ball is placed on the foul line in front of the penalized team's, and a "free kick" is attempted by one of the scorers.
- Goalies stepping over the goal line to make a save will result in a penalty kick for the other team.
- I usually play until a team reaches 10 goals, then a new game is started.
- It is important to use scrimmage vests for easy team recognition.
- Any ball kicked higher than the height restriction on the wall, is not considered a goal, but may be picked up by a goalie and play continues.
- The game is started by rolling the soccer ball between the two scoring groups.
- Encourage scorers not to bunch up, but to stay away from their player with the ball while breaking toward the goal line.

"Knock Down Rotation Kickball"

Grades 2-5
Formation: 2 teams consisting of 3 groups
#1 kicker lines up behind the ball, the rest wait their turn.

#2's are the "fielding team." One fielder is the **"bowler"** (may not step over the bowling line) one fielder is the "retriever" who stands behind the bowling pins, all others are fielders.

Equipment: 1 Kickball, 10 Bowling Pins, 4 Cones, 1 Home Plate.

How to Play:

The kicker kicks the ball and proceeds to run around the cones (1,2,3,4) and return to home plate. The fielder who catches the ball passes it to the bowler. The bowler (without stepping over the line) starts to bowl the ball at the bowling pins. The "retriever" gets the ball back to the bowler as quickly as possible for another try. When the kicker touches home plate, the whistle is blown. The fielding team gets 1 point for every pin knocked down before the whistle blows.

Continued...

Kicking Games

"Knock Down Rotation Kickball"
Continued.......

Rotation:
- Kicker goes to the end of the line.
- A new kicker steps up.
- The bowler becomes the retriever.
- All others rotate as in volleyball.

Tips:
- Gym floor tape makes for a good "bowling line."
- Depending on the kicking skills of the class, the ball may be rolled toward the kicker.
- A cumulative score for the fielding team.

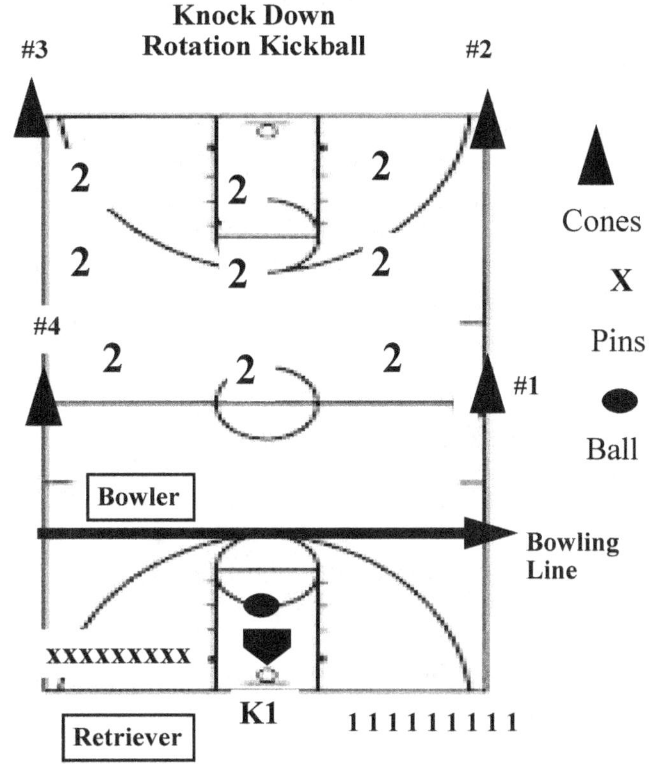

"Kick Pin Defense"
Grades 2-5
Equipment: 1 Kickball, 6 Cones, 1 Bowling Pin per Fielder. 3 Tennis Balls

Formation:
Arrange the fielders into three groups. One group equidistant on the half court line, one group across the foul line, and the last group across the end line. Each fielder stands next to a bowling pin (it is best to place a "poly spot" under each bowling pin to help reset pins quickly).

Starting on the sideline opposite each fielding group, place two cones next to each other with a tennis ball on top of the first cone.

How to Play:
The kicker, upon kicking the ball out into the field starts to run to the first set of cones. Once there, they transfer the tennis ball from cone #1 to cone #2. They then proceed to the second set of cones, and finally the third set. Upon completion, they run straight back and across the finish line. while the kicker is doing the above, , the fielders catch the ball and start passing it to the other fielders who knock their pin down once they catch it. Knock down as many pins as you can until the whistle blows, indicating that the kicker has crossed the finish line. One point is awarded for every pin that gets knocked down.

Rotation:
- The kicker goes to the end of the line, and a new kicker steps up.
- Fielders rotate in a volleyball fashion.
- Switch teams after the last kicker.

Continued...

"Kick Pin Defense"

Tips:
- Have fielders pass the ball to the player closest to them to get as many as possible (i.e. don't throw from the first row to the third, or extreme right or left).

- Any kicked ball that knocks down a pin directly is counted for the "fielding" team.

- Have fielders knock down the pin with the ball while its in their hand rather than throwing it at the pin (this saves time and allows more pins to be knocked down.
  The next kicker will now transfer the pin from the second to the first.

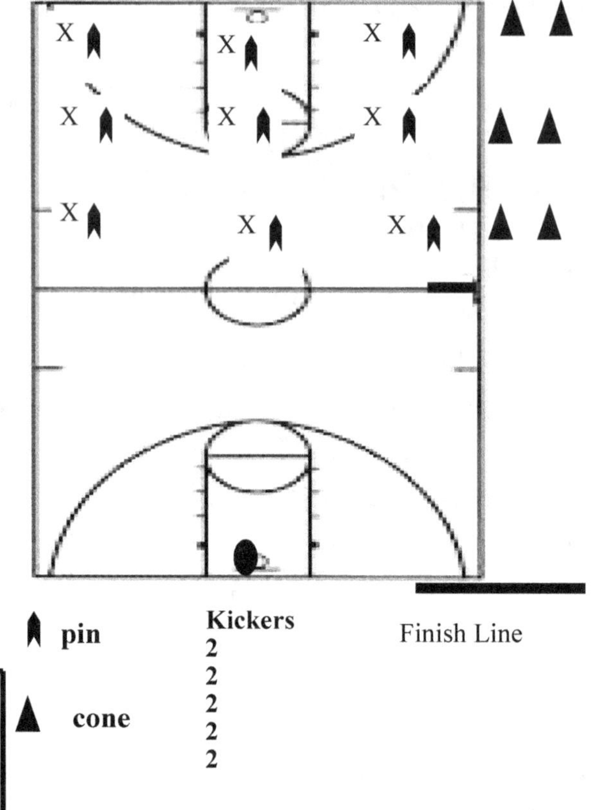

"Kick Pin Kickball"

Grades 2-5

Equipment: 1 Kickball, 4 Bases
Formation:
    One kicker lines up behind the ball, the rest of the kicking team waits their turn. The fielders are spread out in the field (no one in front of the half court line) with 4 fielders next to a pin (in front of 1st, 2nd, and 3rd base, and in front of home plate.

How to Play:
    On the signal "go" the kicker kicks the ball and proceeds to run the basis tagging each. Whoever catches the ball passes it to the closes fielder guarding a pin (does not have to be 1st base). That fielder then will knock the pin down and pass it to the next closest player near a pin. When the kicker touches home plate, the whistle blows. The next kicker steps in and the fielders will keep adding additional pins that are knocked down. (if 3 were knocked down with the first kicker, the next pin will be counted as 4 and so on). After every kicker has kicked once, switch teams, and the new fielding team will try to beat the score of the first team.

Rotation: Rotate in such a way that every fielder covers every spot in the field.

Tips:
- I find numbered poly-spots for all the fielders makes their rotation easier.
- Encourage "direct passes" between fielders.
- The ball can be rolled to a kicker if the skill level allows. A kick that hits a pin counts for the fielding team.

*See Diagram on next page

"Kickpin Kickball" Diagram

Kicking Games

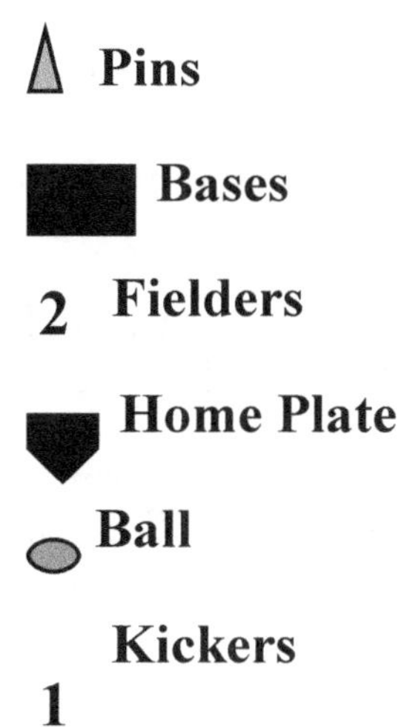

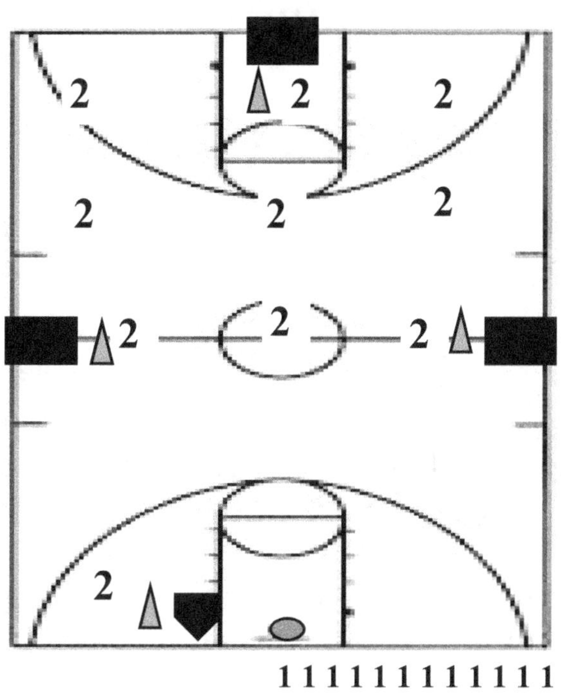

"One on One Kickball"
Grades 2-6

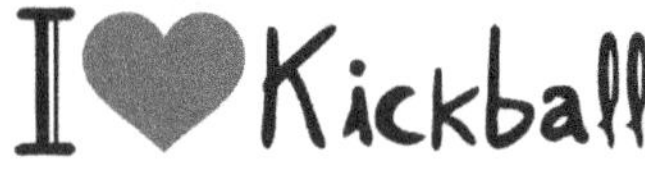

Equipment: 1 Kickball, 4 Bases

Formation:
Two teams, each numbered to establish a rotation order

How to Play:
Team "A" designates player number 1 to field balls within the diamond, remaining players form a line connecting third and home bases. Number 1 of Team "B" stands behind the home plate, and the remaining members of his/her team form a line connecting first and home bases.

The player at home base places the ball on the surface of home plate. Taking one step, they kick the ball and immediately starts around the bases, touching each in turn. The runner tries to reach home base before the fielder secures the ball and returns with it to home plate. As soon as the fielder touches home plate, with the ball in their hand, the runner must stop where they are. The number of bases that they touched are recorded.   their turn is over and they retire to the end position on their team. **Number 2** of the fielding team enters the diamond, and play continues. When each member of Team B has had a turn to kick, a half inning has been completed and Team A gets their turn.

Continued..........

"One on One ..Kickball"
Continued...

Kicking Games

Fly Ball: If a fielder catches a kicked ball before it touches the ground no score is made by the kicker, and another player from each team takes their new position.

Fair Ball: A ball that travels within the area outlined by home plate and first and third bases is a "fair ball."

Second Trial: A player is allowed a second kick if they fail to send the ball within the boundaries on the first try. On a second failure, their turn is finished and they retire to the end position of their team.

Scoring: The kicking team scores one point for each base reached before the fielder contacts home plate, as follows: 1 point when first base is reached; 2 points second base; 3 points third base, 4 points, home base.

The team having the highest number of points at the end of the agreed upon number of innings is the winner.

Tips:
- Have the kicker focus their eyes on the ball until their foot contacts it.
- Have children manage their own game by stationing a child with a whistle behind home plate to signal whenever a fielder touches it. The runner stops at the whistle, and the number of bases they have touched is recorded.

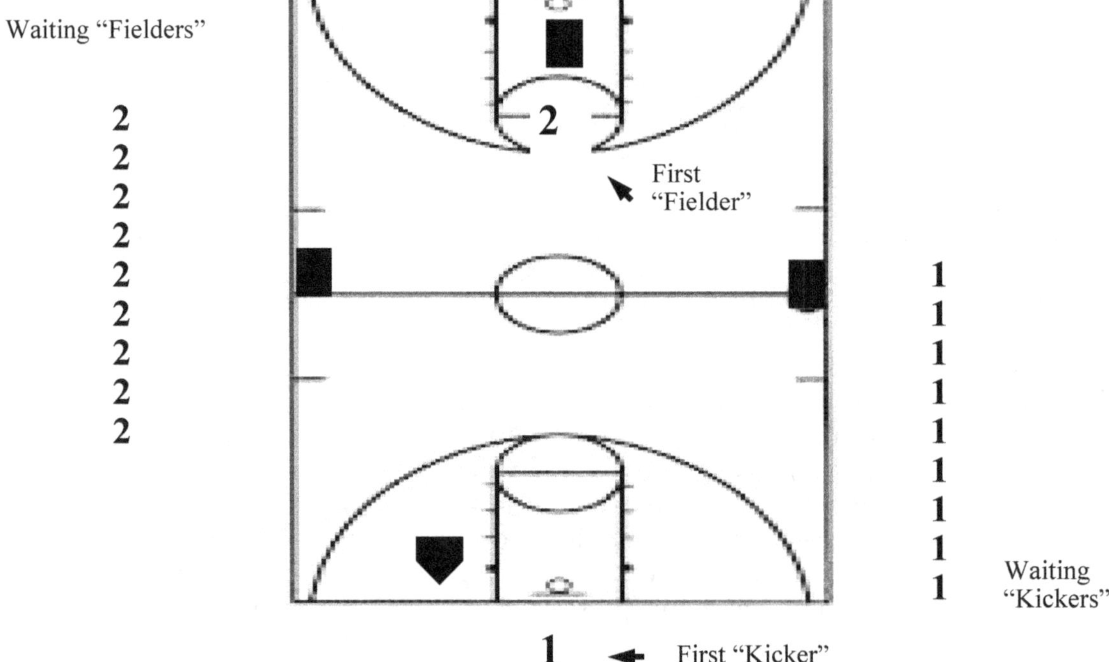

"One on One ..Kickball"
With A Catcher.......

Kicking Games

Always play this game <u>after</u> "One on One Kickball"

In this game the fielder, upon catching the ball, throws to their catcher who steps on home. Same scoring rules apply. This is a good game to reinforce strong accurate throws.

Rotation: Catcher becomes fielder, fielder goes to the end of the line, next fielder becomes the catcher.

KICKBALL

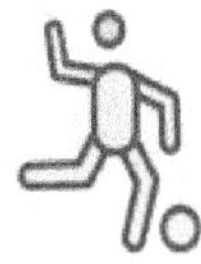 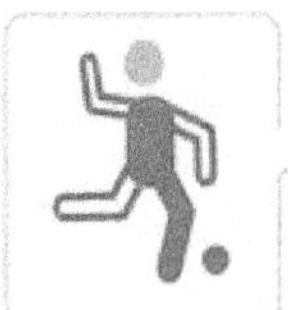 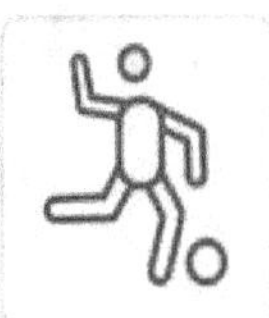 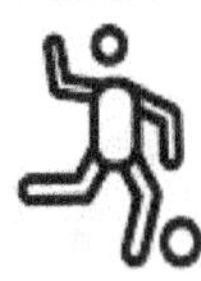 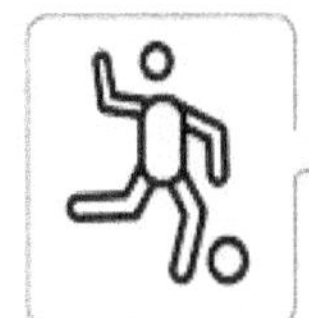 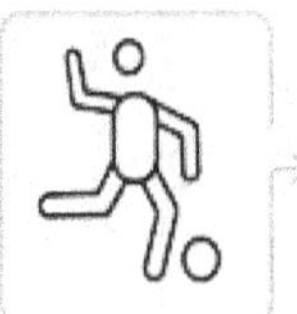

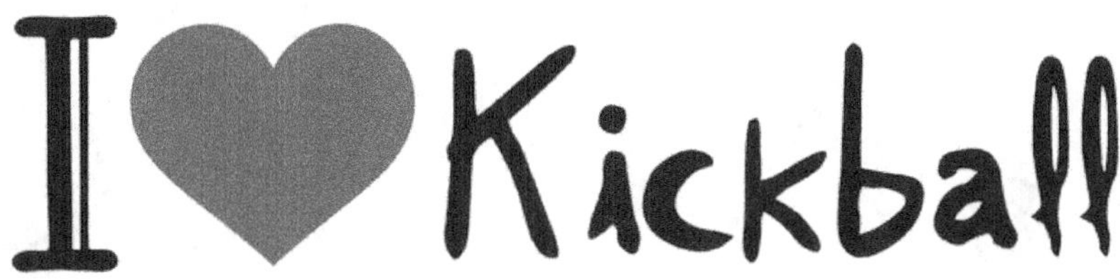

Jim Eagan

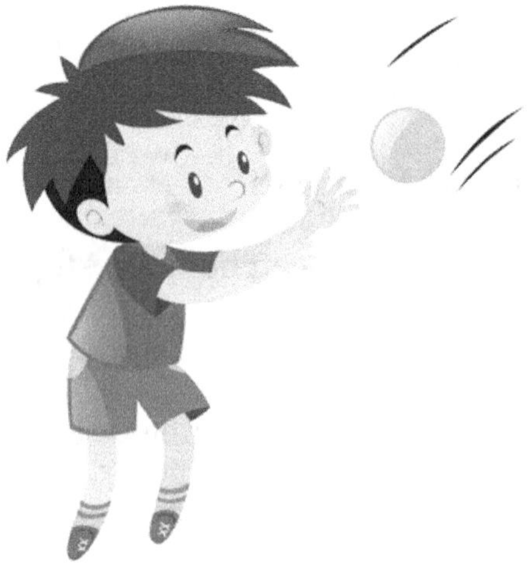

Throwing & Catching Games

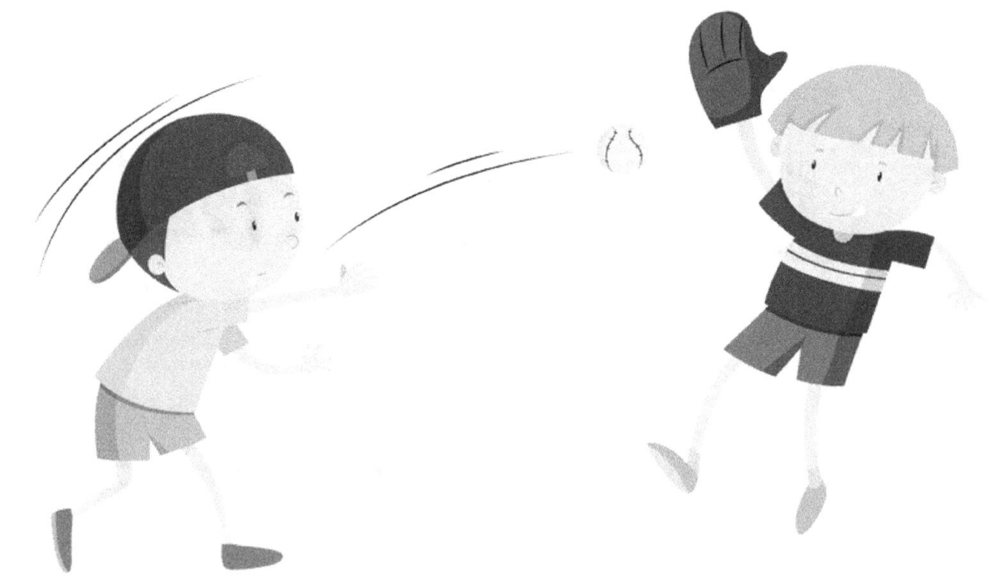

Throwing and Catching Games

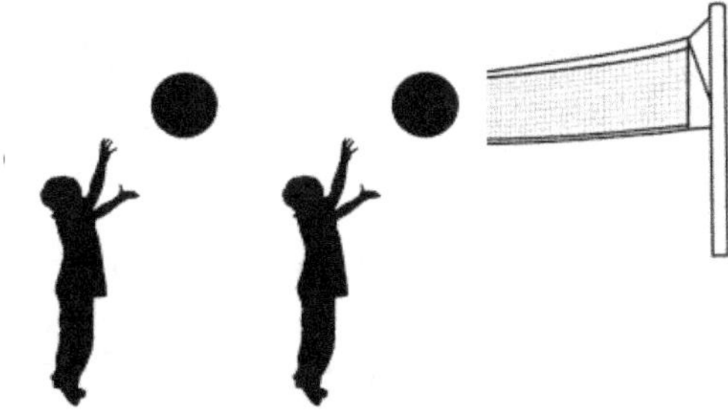

"Sock, It To Me"

Grade Level: K-6
Equipment: 1 Ball per child, Volleyball net
Formation: One team scattered on each side of the net.

How to Play:

When the starting signal is given, everyone will throw their ball over the net and throw back any that come from the other team as fast as they can. This will continue until the whistle is heard. No balls may be thrown after this time. The team with the fewest balls on its side wins.

Tip: It is best to use 6 inch "Nerf" or "soft coated balls. For K-2 students: lower net to 4 feet.

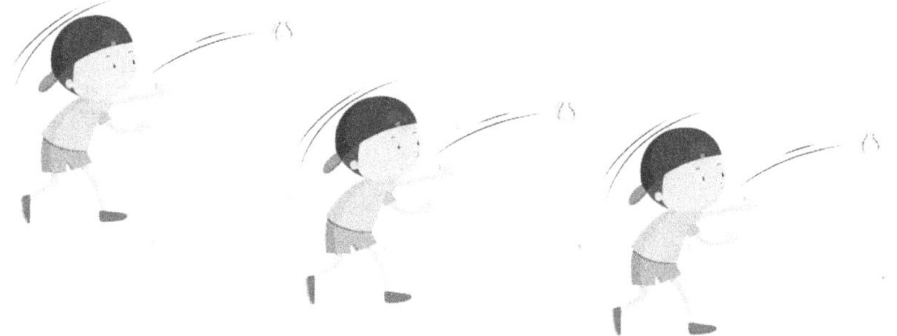

"Throw and Go"

Grade Level: K-3
Equipment: A distinguishable ball and a starting mark for each team.
Formation: Teams are lined up in file formation.

How to Play:

The first player on each team holds a ball and stands on their mark. When the signal is given, player throws the ball as straight and as far as possible. They then run to retrieve any ball other than their own and bring it back to their line. First team back with a different ball scores 1 point for the team.

Tip: This is a great game to develop "distance throwing skills" using the basic learning concepts of throwing skills.

"Double Trouble" | Throwing and Catching Games

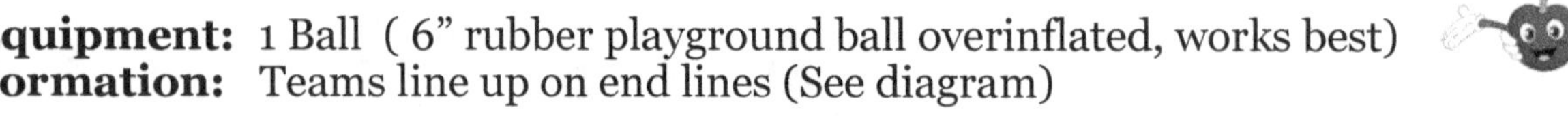

Grade Level: K-3

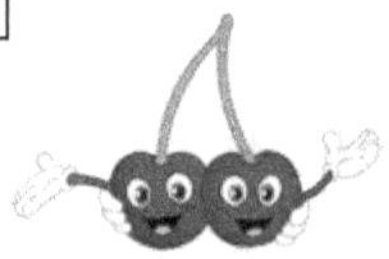

Equipment: 1 Ball (6" rubber playground ball overinflated, works best)
Formation: Teams line up on end lines (See diagram)

How to Play:
Teacher stands in the center and starts play by tossing the ball vertically (overhead), calling out any number, and quickly steps out of the way. The object of the game is for all players (whose number was called) to try to catch the ball. The one who succeeds scores a point for their team and returns to their original starting spot. The teacher calls another number. The team that scores a predetermined number designated by the teacher at the start wins.

Modification: Teacher can vary the type of throw, or timing when calling the number called to add variety.

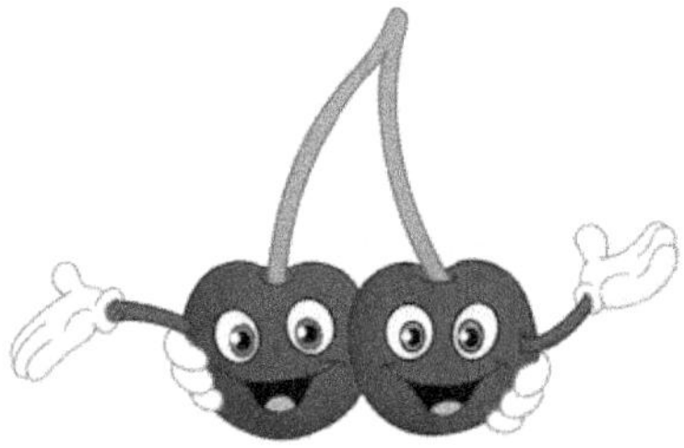

"Double Trouble"

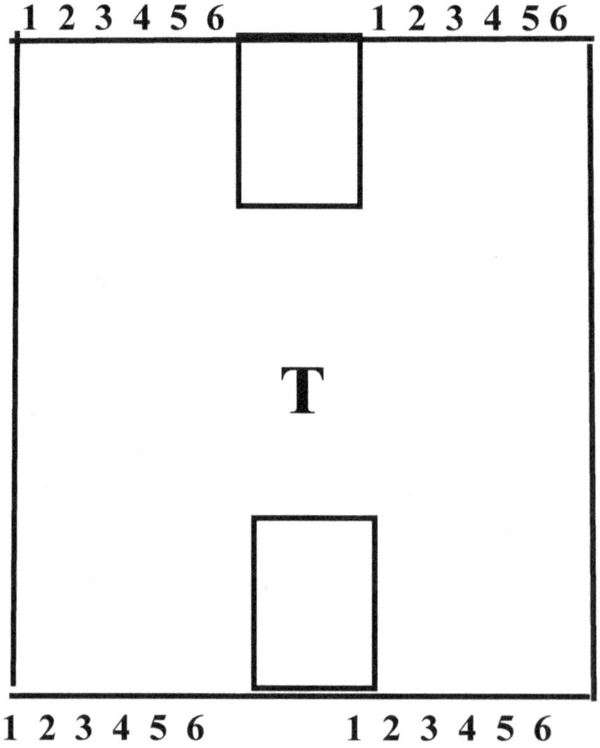

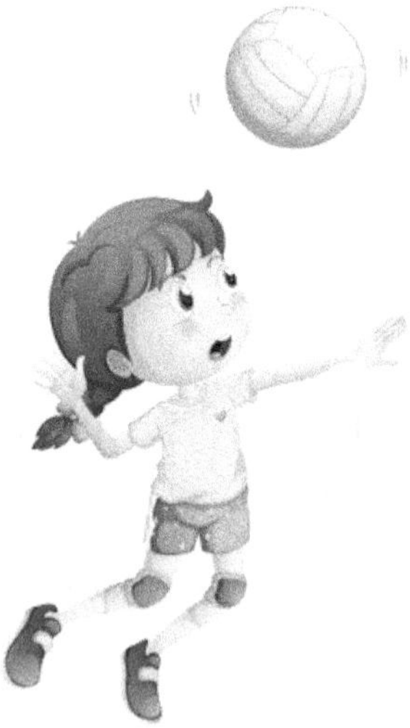

1 2 3 4 5 6   1 2 3 4 5 6

T

1 2 3 4 5 6   1 2 3 4 5 6

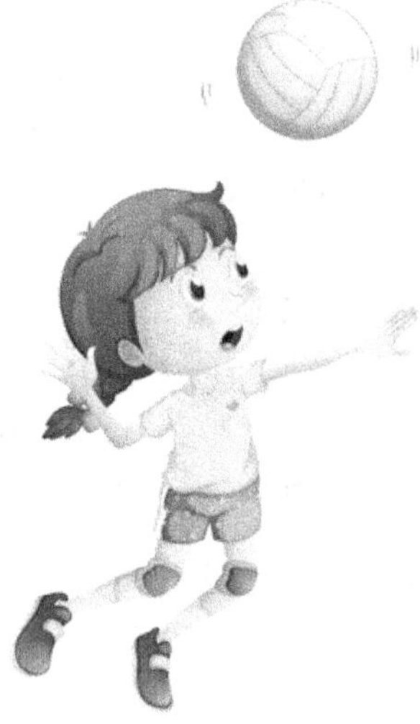

Throwing and Catching Games

"Stop Thief"

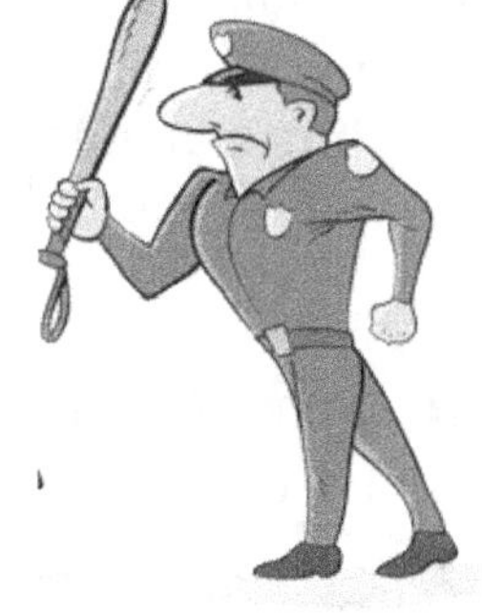

Grade Level: K– 6
Equipment: 1 Ball - 6" to 8" , One bowling pin or beanbag.
Formation: 2 lines 40' apart.

How to Play:

Each player is given a number and stands on his or her team's line. The teacher then selects one team to be the runners, the other as throwers. The teacher then calls out a number. The players with that number come out, the runners go for the pin, the throwers for the ball. **Scoring:** 1 point for the runners if they can carry the pin across the goal line, 2 points for throwers if they hit the runners before they reach the goal line. After all numbers are called , teams switch roles.

Suggestion: Place both ball and pin the same distance from each end line.

Tip: This is a fun game that kids really enjoy. However, in keeping with the philosophy of more students being involved at any one time, I divide the gym up into three games running simultaneously. The teacher controls play by starting each round on a whistle. When playing with grades k-2, I will move the end lines in closer, and further away for the grade 3-6 students. Also, I encourage the "throwers" to run a few steps then **"Stop, Aim, and Throw."**

Runners

B1 B2 B3 B4   C1 C2C3 C4

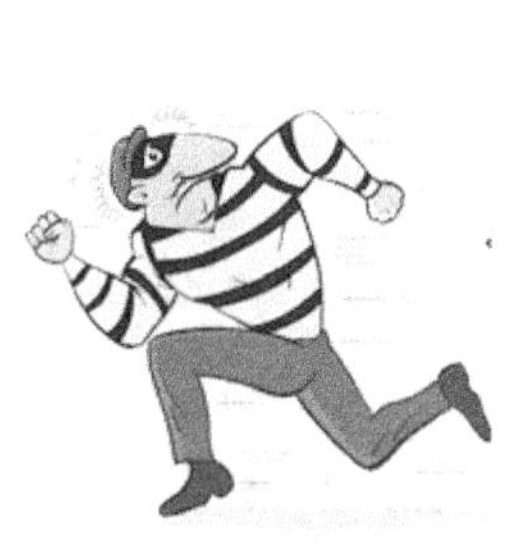

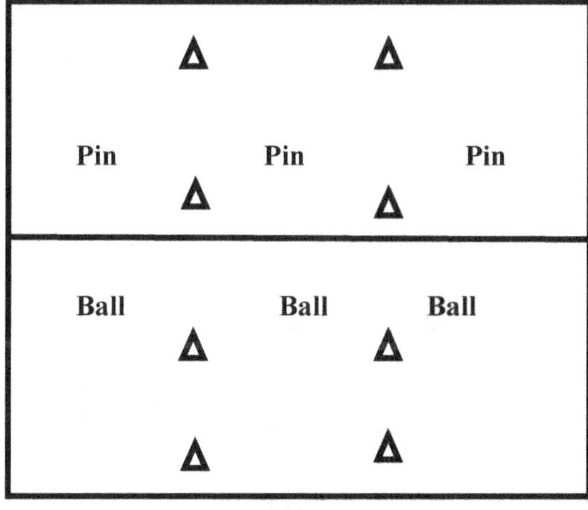

A1 A2 A3 A4

Throwers

"Pin Pass" | Throwing and Catching Games |

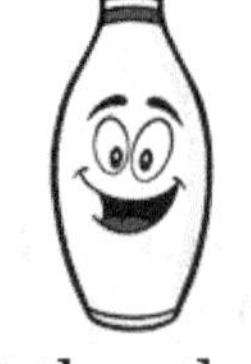

Grade Level: K– 6

Equipment: 3 Balls, 3 Bowling Pins

Formation: 3 teams, 1 thrower who starts with a ball facing their partner. At the other end of the gym, standing behind a bowling pin.

How to Play:

We usually play this game after having taught and practiced the correct way to throw and catch.

On the signal "go", throwers 1,2, and 3 throw the ball across the gym to their partner. The "catcher," upon catching the ball taps their pin down with the ball (don't throw the ball). Give a point to the first two teams that knock down their pins.

Rotation: The catchers will pick up the pins and become the throwers, and the throwers will become the catchers. Once everyone has had a chance, bring in a new set of players.

Tip: Explain that the more accurate you are with your throws, the better chance your partner will be first or second to knock the pin down. A crooked throw will make your partner waste time running to the pin after catching the ball.

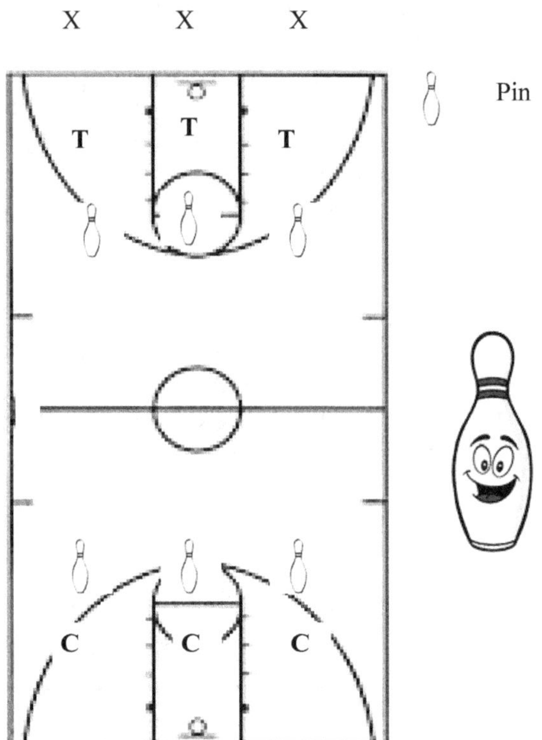

"Double Pin Pass"

To make the game more challenging, try this twist. When the catcher knocks down the pin, they now have to throw it back and the original thrower knocks down their pin also. Again, the first two teams to knock down both pins score a point.

Rotation: the next two players on each team step in and the catcher and thrower go to the end of their team's line.

Sometimes the second throw is rushed and poor form occurs. Explain that its better to take an extra second to get in the throwing position then to hurry and make a poor throw.

"Guard the Castle"

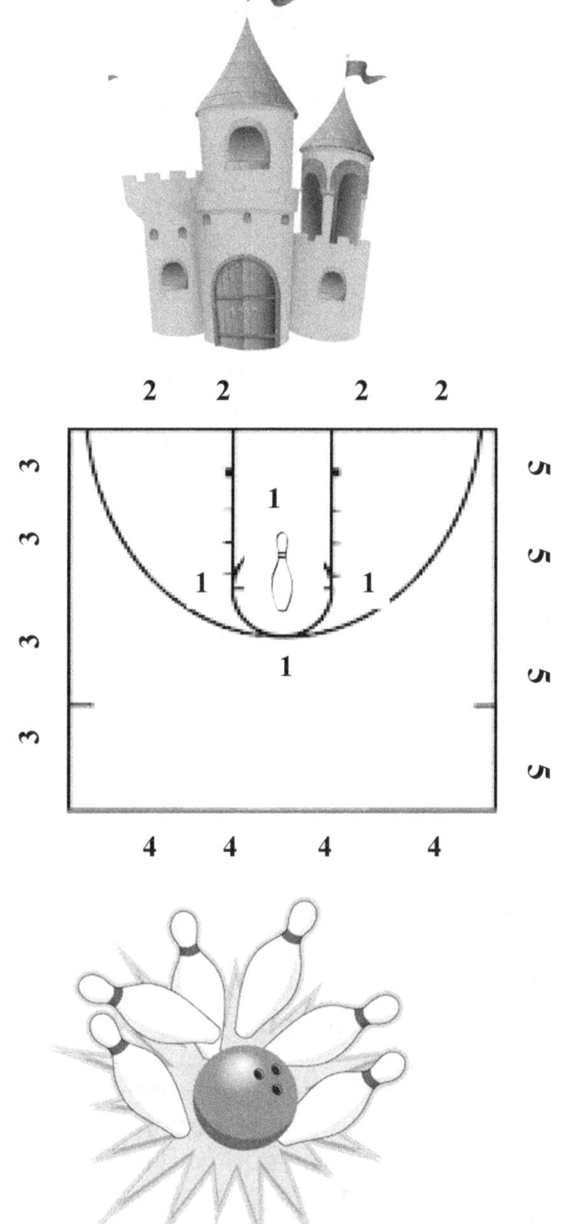

Throwing and Catching Games

Grade Level: K– 5

Equipment: 1 bowling pin, and 1 ball for each of the players on the throwing teams.

Formation: 5 Teams—4 Teams using 1/4 of the 1/2 court, and 1 team blocking the bowling pin.

How To Play: The four blockers (who are not allowed to step in the area between the foul line and the top of the circle) attempt to keep the pin up for the maximum 30 seconds. They can block throws by batting balls, kicking balls, or whatever it takes to keep the pin up.

The other teams are throwing the balls in an attempt to knock the pin down. Additional throws may be made if they are able to get a ball without stepping over the line. The instructor signals "go" and starts the stopwatch. Blow the whistle if (1) 30 seconds have elapsed, (2) when the pin is knocked down. Score 1 point for every second you can keep the pin standing (blockers) a maximum of 30 points. After 30 seconds rotate another throwing team in, and move the blockers to one of the throwing areas. Throwing teams also rotate clockwise until it is their turn to block.

"Pin Bombardment"

Grade Level: 1– 5

Formation: 2 Teams: A and B. Half of each team are "throwers" who cannot step over half court. The other half are "throwers " who cannot step over the end line. Five bowling pins are positioned equidistant half way between the half court and end line. Ideally, each player should have a ball.

Continued on next page......

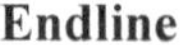

Throwing and Catching Games

Pin Bombardment

"Pin Bombardment" Cont.

How To Play: On the signal "go", everyone starts throwing (overhand or bowling) the balls attempting to knock down pins that they are facing. Continue until one team knocks down all five, at which point the whistle blows and a point is awarded.

To start the next round, have all the pins picked up and once everyone has retrieved a ball, have the half-court throwers become the end line throwers, and vice-versa.

Tip: Explain that if one of the half-court throwers wants to block a pin, they may, but only one person may block a pin. Another modification is to place the pins inside hoops—this makes it more challenging for a blocker who cannot step inside the hoop.

"End Ball"

Grade Level: 3–5

Equipment: Enough balls for every thrower on both teams to start with.

Formation: Divide each team into 3 equal groups. One group are *catchers* (they are stationed between the end wall of the gym and the end line, which they cannot cross). Another group are the *throwers* (they are not allowed to cross the half court line when throwing). The final group are the *defenders* (they are not allowed to step over the line into the "catcher's" area

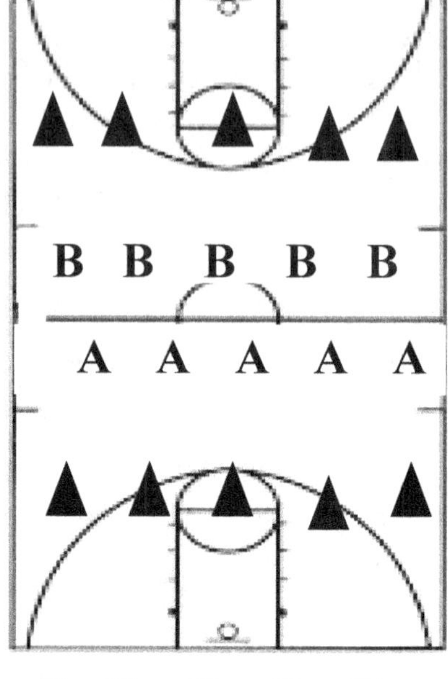

End Ball

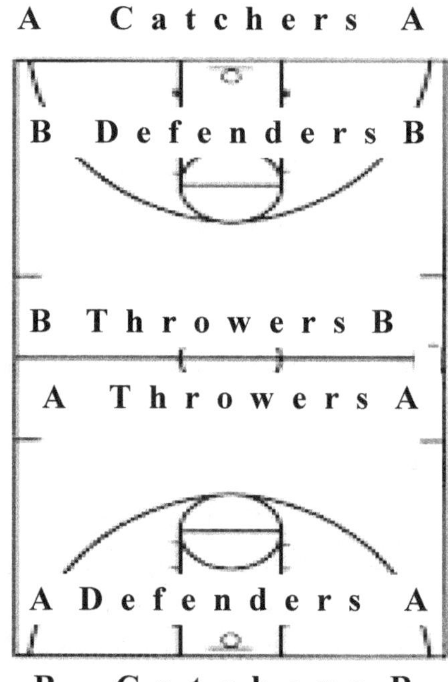

Continued on next page………

"End Ball"
Continued...

Throwing and Catching Games

How To Play:

On the signal **"go,"** the **throwers** attempt to throw the ball to their **catchers.** The **defenders**, without stepping over the end line, attempt to block or intercept the throws. Every time a catcher is successful catching the ball (it must be on a fly) they are finished and step out of bounds. Play continues until all the catchers are finished and that team scores the point. To start the next round teams rotate the following way: Throwers become catchers, catchers become defenders, and defenders become throwers.

Tip: When a **defender** intercepts a ball, have them throw it to their <u>throwers</u> instead of throwing the ball to their <u>catchers</u> themselves.

"Freedom Ball"
Grade Level: 3– 5

Equipment: At least one ball for every other thrower if not more (the more the better**)**.

Formation: Divide the team into 2 groups. Group 1 are the "throwers, and they are allowed to move about from half court to the end line, without crossing either line. Group 2 are the 'catchers" and they must stay between the wall and the end line.

How To Play:

On the signal **"go"** the **throwers** start throwing to their **catchers**.
When a catcher catches a ball in the air, they are allowed to leave the catching area and join the throwers. They must bring the ball with them. The game continues until all the "catchers" are "freed" from their area. One point is then awarded to that team. Catchers and throwers switch places at the conclusion of each round.

Tip: When leaving the catching area, leave by running up the sideline as indicated in the diagram. This will avoid collisions with the other team. Balls that get stuck by the half court line and end line may be picked up by any thrower.

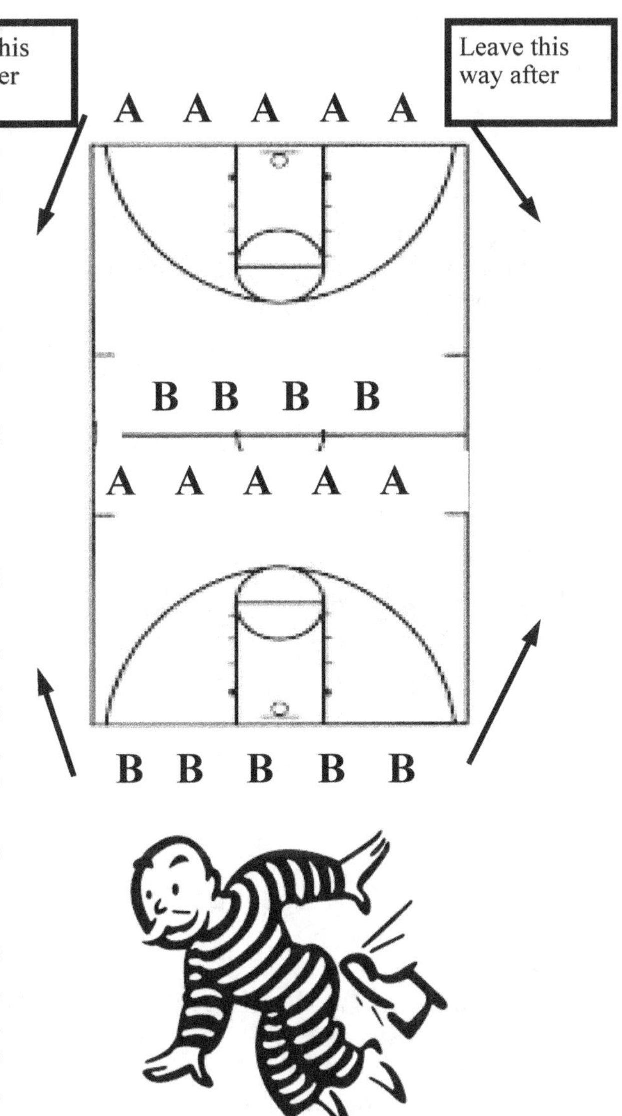

Throwing and Catching Games

"Basketball Target Throw"

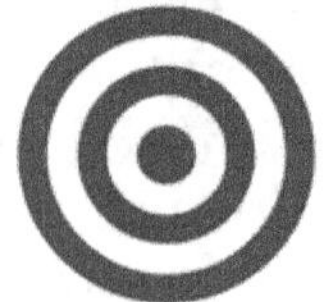 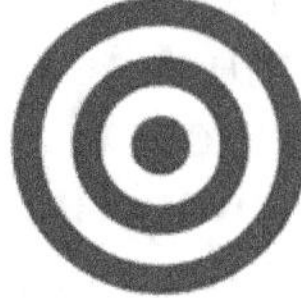 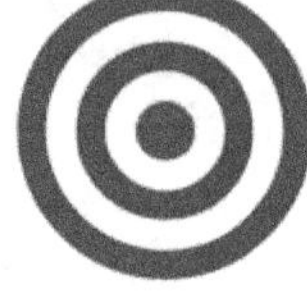

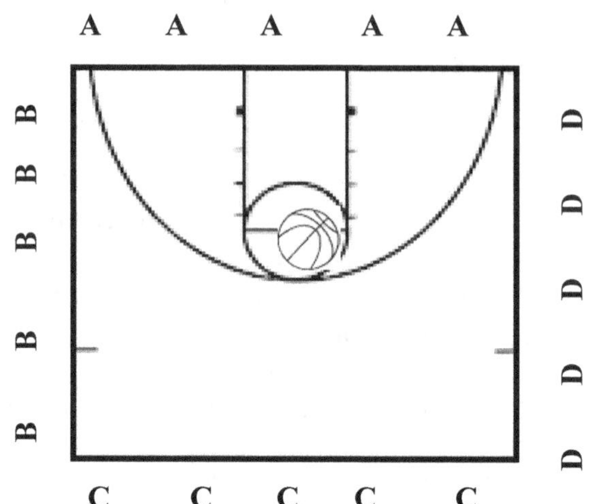

Grade Level: 1– 5

Equipment: One basketball placed on the foul line, and one 6" playground ball for every player.

Formation: 4 Teams (each team covering 1/4 of the half court.)

How To Play:
On the signal "go" players on all four teams attempt to throw the playground balls at the basketball causing it to cross one of the other team's line. Play continues until the basketball crosses one of the lines. At this point the instructor blows the whistle and awards a point to every team except the one that let the ball cross their line. To start the next game, everyone gets a ball, the basketball is placed in the middle, and play continues.

Tip: To start the next game, have teams rotate one line to the right so they all get a chance to throw from different positions. Stress that the only way to save the ball from crossing their line is by throwing a ball. If they touch it with their body or kick it, the whistle blows and the ball is considered crossing their team's line.

"Water Sprite with a Ball"

Grade Level: K-2

Equipment: One ball (Tagger has a ball)

Formation: Same as "Water Sprite" (See Water Sprite in Movement Section)

How To Play:
Same as "Water Sprite" (See Movement Section) except that instead of tagging one of the four runners, players attempt to hit them with a thrown ball.

Tip: At first you may allow the thrower to chase one of the four players to hit them with the ball. To make it more challenging, do not allow them to leave the semi-circle to throw in an attempt to hit a runner.

Throwing and Catching Games

"Guard the Castle <u>Full Court</u>"

Grade Level: 2– 5
Equipment: A ball For Each Player, 4 Pins, 4 Hoops.
Formation: 2 teams. Both teams have throwers that start behind the sidelines and end lines. **<u>The half court line is not used.</u>** 3 players from each team act as "blockers" who attempt to keep the 2 pins from falling.

How To Play: Connect 2 hoops and place them on each foul line. Put a bowling pin inside each hoop. Each blocker is responsible for the throwers that they are facing. On the signal "go" throwers attempt to knock down the pins, while the blockers attempt to block balls any way they can. When one team has knocked down both of the opponent's pins, the instructor blows the whistle ending play. The team with pins still standing gets a point for each one not knocked down.

Rotation: The blockers go back to their team and three new players become blockers.

Tips:
- No throwers are allowed to step over the end or sideline to get another ball. They may throw another ball if it crosses their line only.

- Encourage blockers to catch a ball instead of kicking them. Kicking it will give the other team more opportunities. Any ball caught may be thrown to a member of the blocking team by the blocker.

- No one should be hit in the face with a ball, since all throws will be thrown low to knock over a pin.

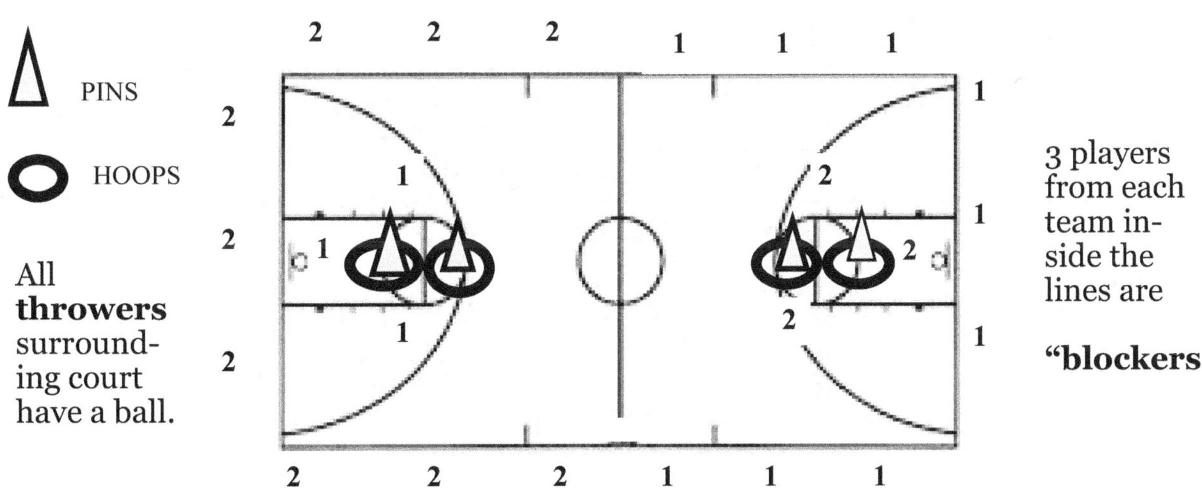

Throwing and Catching

" Progressive Bowling"

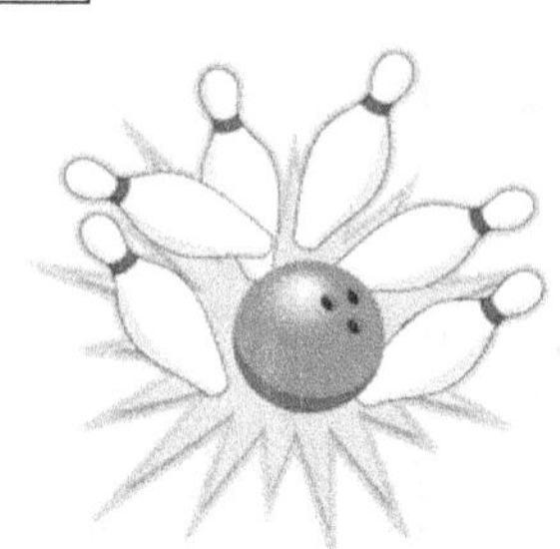

Grade Level: 2– 5

Equipment: 4 bowling pins, 4 6" Playground Balls, 12 Poly Spots.

Formation:
- 4 "Bowlers" starting behind the half court line.
- 4 'Chasers" standing behind the first bowling pin.
- 4 Lines of players who are next.

How To Play:
On the signal, the first 4 players <u>bowl</u> the ball toward the pin on the first spot. When the pin gets knocked down, it is placed on the second spot. If it doesn't get knocked down, it stays on that spot. The first team to knock the pins down from all 3 spots gets a point. Pins are brought back to the first spot and the game continues.

Rotation: The **bowler** is responsible for putting a knocked down pin on the next spot. If the bowler doesn't knock down the pin, they simply become the **"chaser'**. The chaser is responsible for bringing the ball back to the next bowler (who has stepped up to the starting line).

Tip: Have bowlers start at least one step behind the starting line so they don't step over it.

Chasers

**Pins
In Polyspots**

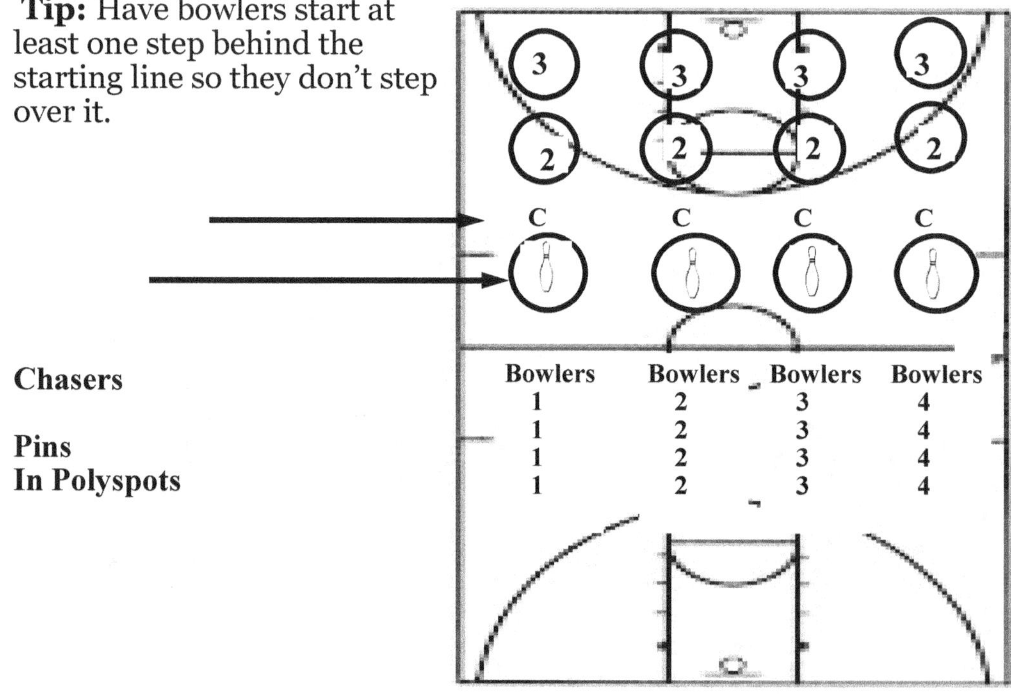

Throwing and Catching Games

"Alley Ball"

Grade Level: K-2

Equipment: 4 cones, 1 ball for each "thrower."

Formation: 3 teams:
#1's the running team.   First runner behind the starting line, all others wait their turn in line.
#2 and **3's** are the throwing teams with each thrower having a ball and standing on each sideline.

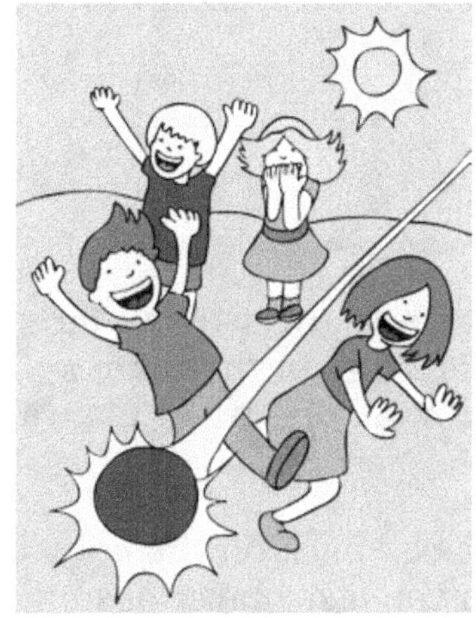

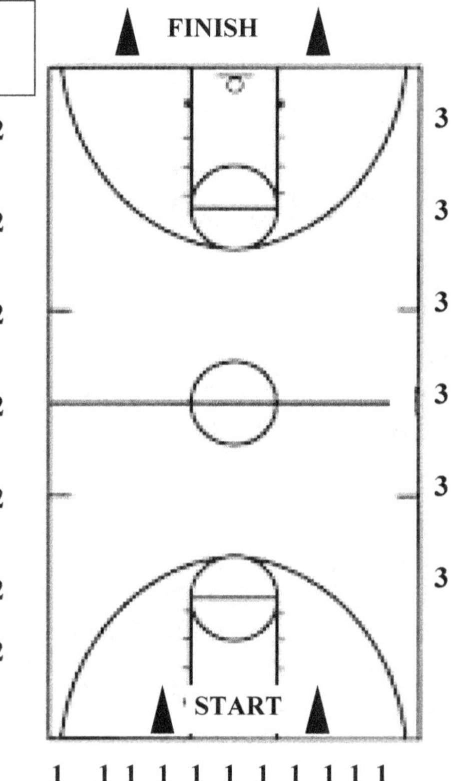

How To Play:
On the signal "go" the runner runs to the finish line. They <u>do not</u> stop when hit by a ball, however you must remind them to remember how many balls hit them. The throwers throw the ball when the runner gets across from them.. When the runner crosses the finish line have them tell you how many times they were hit. The next runner will step in. At this time **the throwers retrieve any ball and go back to their spot and continue**. Once everyone on the running team has had a turn, they reverse direction and start at the finish line and run back to the starting line. Have the running team replace one of the throwing teams and continue until every team has had a chance to run.

Tip: No thrower is allowed to step across the sideline to get a ball. If a ball crosses the sideling they may pick it up for a second throw. A more challenging way to play this game is to have the runner cross the finish line and then return back to the start on each turn. This allows throwers to possibly get a second chance to throw.

Throwing and Catching Games

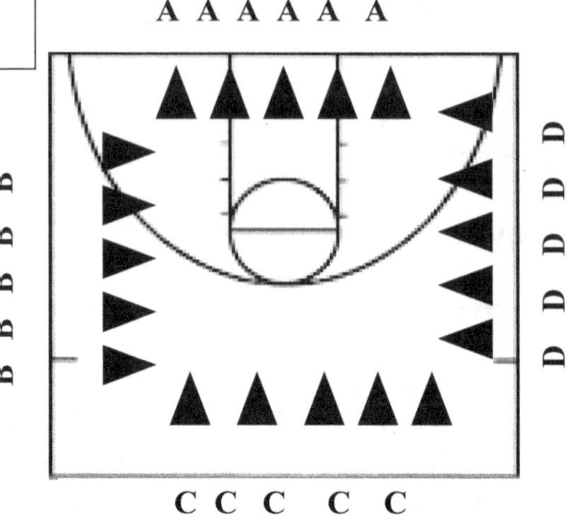

"4 Team Pin Ball"

Grade Level: 1-5

Equipment: 20 bowling Pins, 1 ball for each person, poly-spots for each pin placement.

Formation:
- 4 teams: each team lines up on one of the 1/2 court sidelines.

- 5 bowling pins placed in front of each team (Pins are placed 6 to 10 feet in front of each team and spaced 1 foot apart).

How To Play:
On the signal "go", each team attempts to throw (over or underhand) at any of the **other** team's pins. The game continues until one of the team's pins have all been knocked down, at which point the whistle blows. One point is awarded to the other three teams that still have pins standing.

Rotation: To start the next game, all pins are placed back on the poly-spots, everyone gets a ball, and each rotates to the right with the last player assuming the first position.

Tip: Teams should try to knock down the pins of the teams to the right or left first (these are the closest) before attempting to hit the pins across from them. Also, no one is allowed to step over the sideline to retrieve a ball. Balls crossing the line may be picked up and thrown. Balls that don't cross the line must remain there till the end of the round.

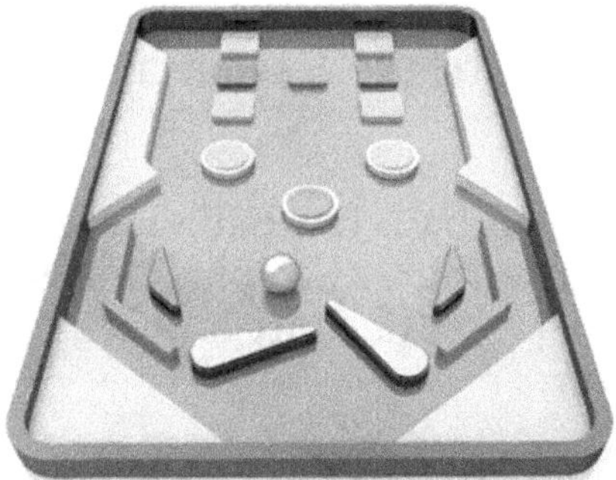
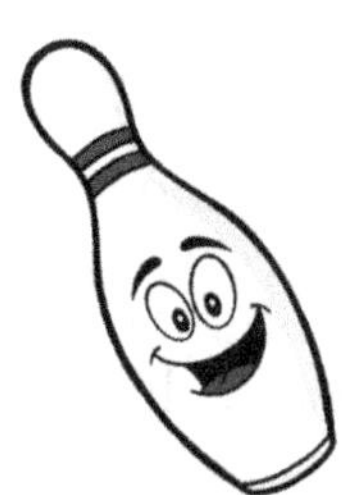
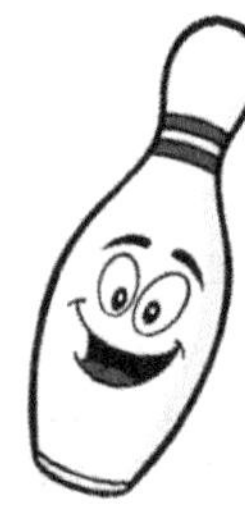
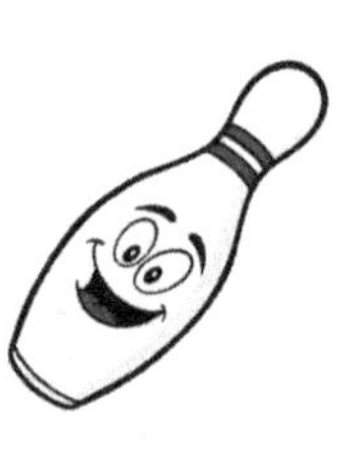

"Castle Ball"
"The Series"

Throwing and Catching

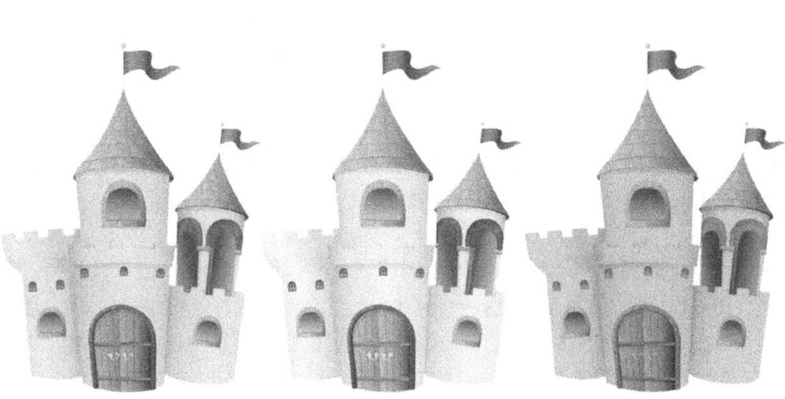

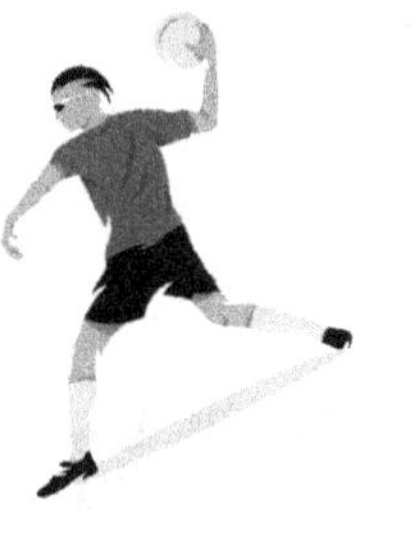

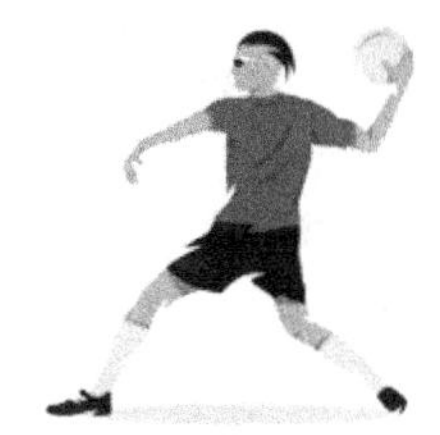

"Castle Ball"

Is a game that students would play every day if you gave them a choice. It is that much fun!! I would like to credit my nephew, Matt Caione, an Elementary Physical Education teacher in the Carmel N.Y. School District, for telling me about this great game. All of the variations of this game are based on the building, destruction, and rebuilding of the "Hula Hoop" castles.

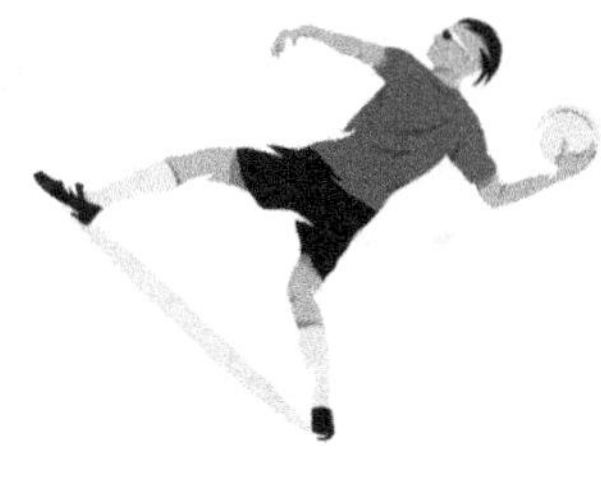

Jim

Building The Castle

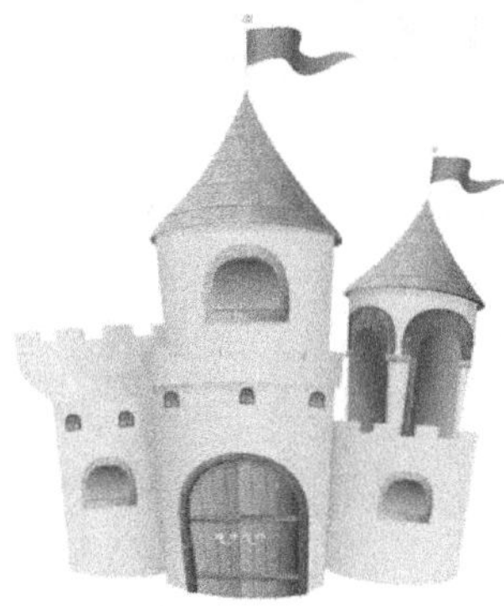

A "Castle" is formed by 6 hula hoops. The first hoop is placed on the ground representing the floor. The next 4 hoops make up the "walls" that are placed inside the floor, two at a time. Once all 4 walls are up, the "roof" is gently place on top securing the castle.

Continued..............

"Castle Ball" continued

Throwing and Catching

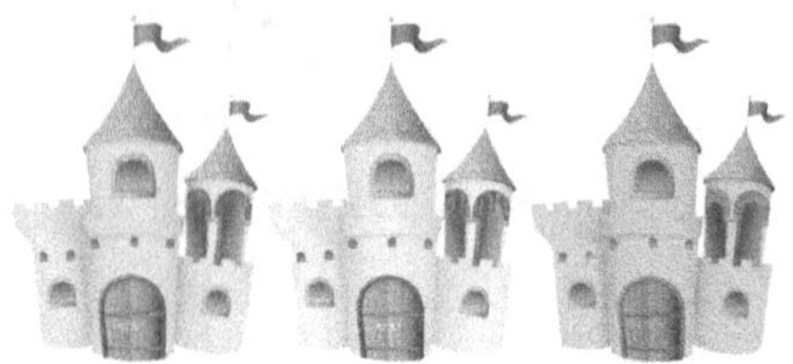

Grade Level: 2-5
Equipment: 1 ball for Each "Thrower",
6 hoops For Each "Castle"

"Games that can be played are limitless." Feel free to be creative. The following are some of the games that have worked well for me:

The first time I introduce **"Castle Ball"** the class will come into the gym where I have already spread out the hoops in piles of 6. There are six piles for each group. I then demonstrate to the class how a castle is made (this really intrigues them). I emphasize the fact that teamwork is essential. Three (3) students per castle works the best (#1 is responsible for the floor and roof, #'s 2 & 3 work on the walls). **Working in groups of 3, I give them 5 minutes or so to practice the construction of the "castle."**

In the first game I play I have the groups on the signal "go" construct a castle as quickly as possible. After a few practice rounds, I eliminate the last group to construct their "castle" each round until one group is left and declared the winner. This activity usually takes a full period. At the end of this session, I explain to the class that the next time we meet we will be using balls to try to knock down the "castles" of the opposing teams.

"Castle Knockdown" (refer to diagram on next page)

The castles are all built and spread out equidistantly along the foul line extended. Every **"thrower"** from each team starts with a ball. Throwers cannot cross the half court line while throwing. **"retrievers"** start behind the castles and get any ball thrown by their own team that passes the castles, and then throw them back to their throwers for another try. The game continues until one team has knocked down all of the other team's castles. The whistle will indicate that one team has won, and now all the castles that have been knocked down get rebuilt and the throwers will now become retrievers, and the retrievers become throwers for the next round of play. Play continues until one team has 5 points. Play as many **5** point games as time allows.

As the class is ready to leave, make sure that you let them know that if they thought today's activity was fun, just wait until next time when they will be playing "Castle Knockdown Rebuild" **I guarantee you will see the excitement on their faces!!"**

Tip: Stress that at no time can throwers block their castle. The penalty for blocking a castle is that it automatically must get knocked down (the teacher should do this to avoid chaos). Any balls that get stuck between half court and the castles must be picked up by a thrower since the retrievers may not come in front of their team's castles. Explain to the throwers not to attempt a throw from where they pick up the ball, but to get closer to the half court line before they throw.

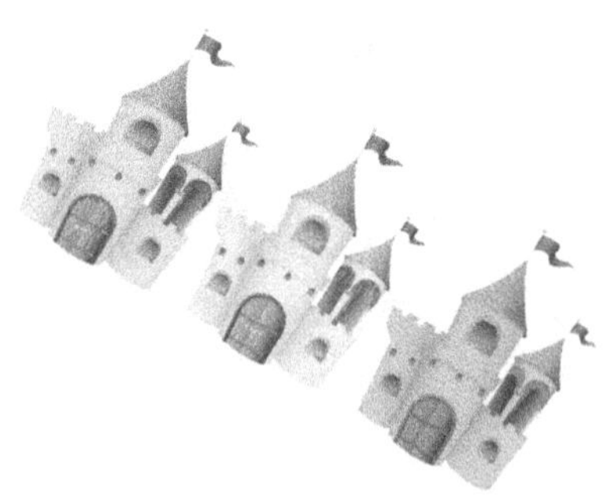

"Castle Knockdown Rebuild"

Throwing and Catching

This is the third activity in Castle ball, and without a doubt the most challenging. Teamwork is essential in this game.

How to Play:

Everything is the same as "Castle Knockdown with one exception. When the whistle blows indicating a winner, all the castles that have been knocked down are to

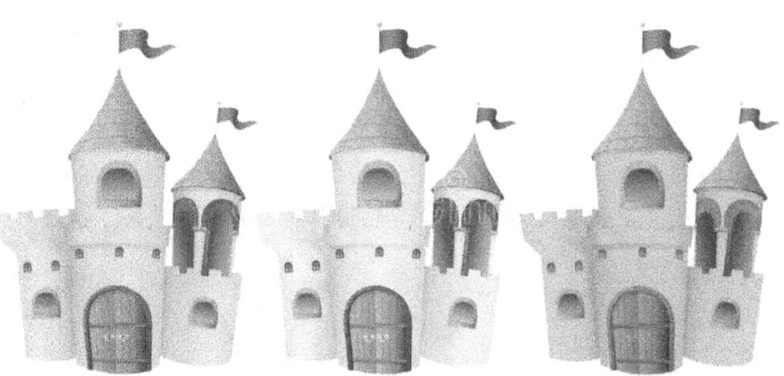

be rebuilt as quickly as possible. The team that has all of their castles built first scores a point. So two points are awarded. One for knocking down all of the castles of your opponent first, and one point for being the first team to rebuild all of your knocked down castles.

Here's where teamwork really pays off. When rebuilding the castles, work as a group (groups of three work best). These groups of 3 can be predetermined before the game begins.

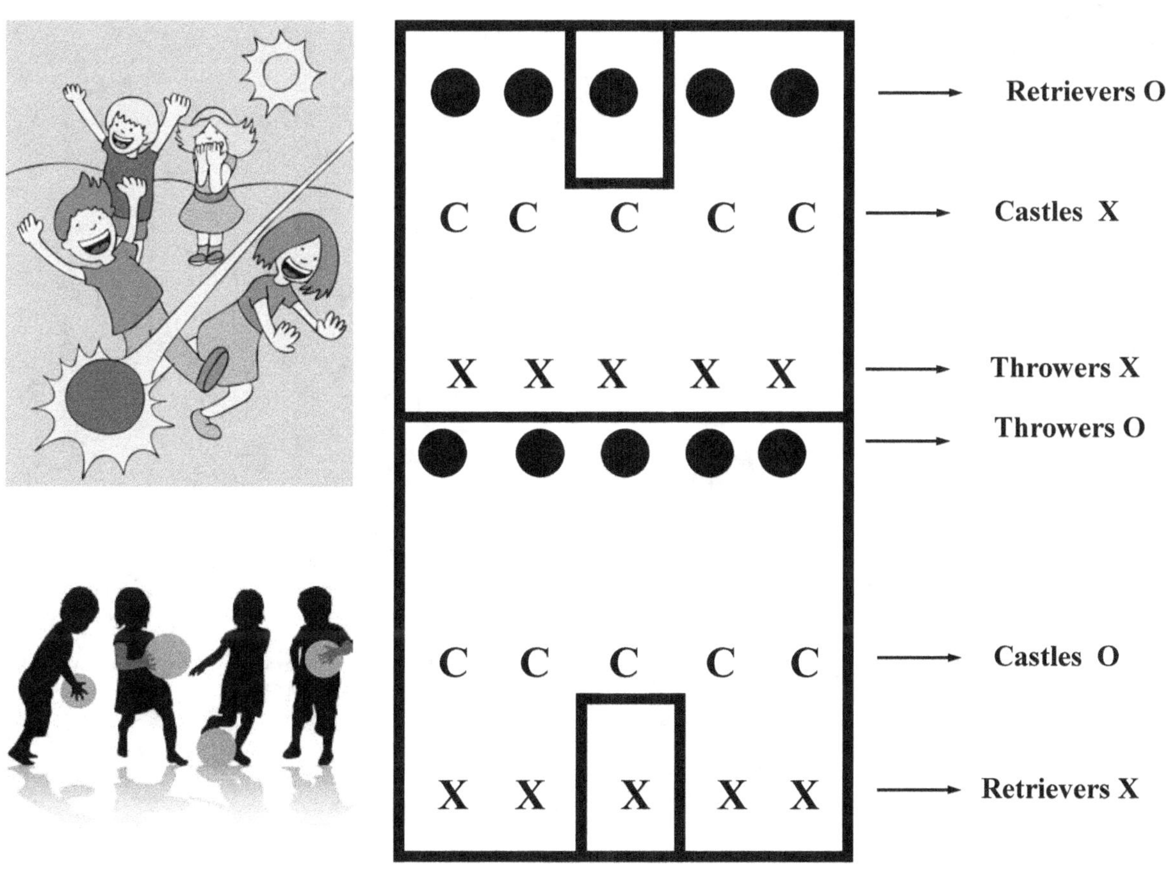

Basketball Games

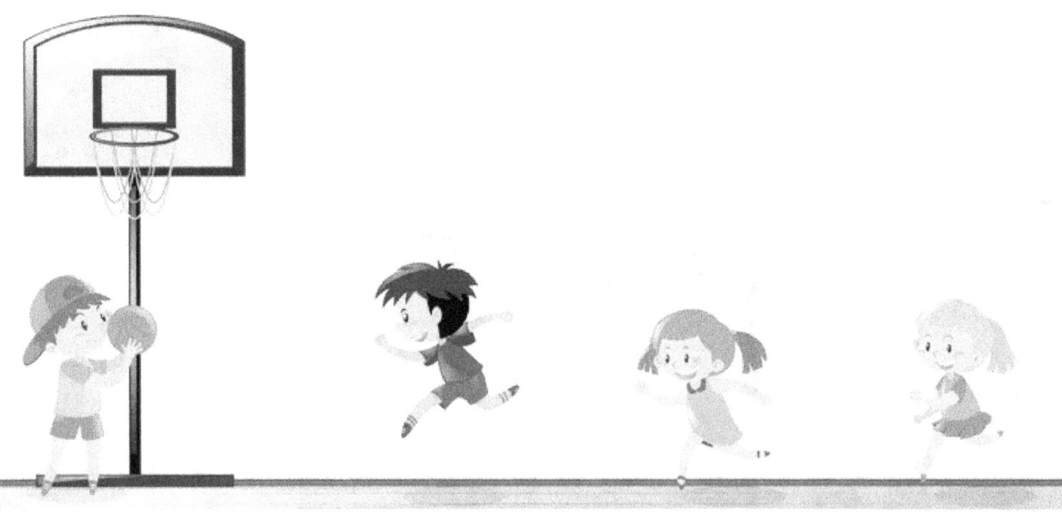

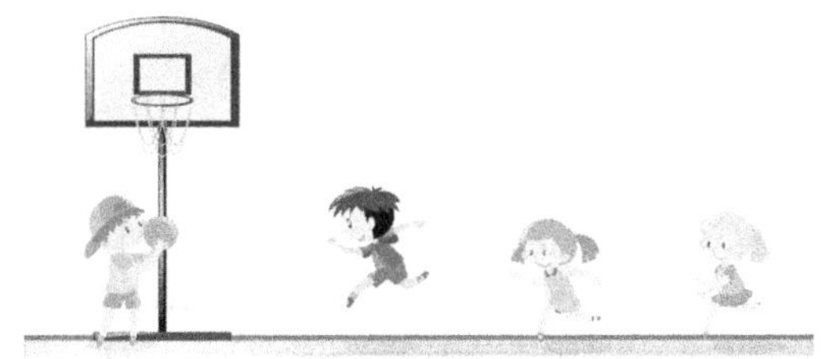

"Basketball Layups"

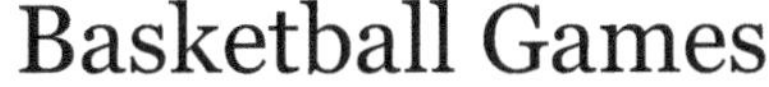

Basketball Games

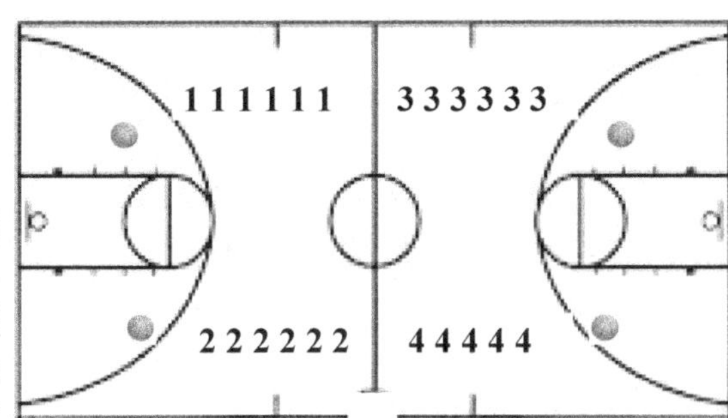

When starting a basketball unit, it is important to emphasize the following skills: Dribbling, Layup Shooting, and Passing.

Grades 3-5
Formation: 4 equal teams, 2 at each basket
Equipment: 4 Basketballs

How to Play:
    This is the first activity that I use when I start a basketball unit. It is a great way to emphasize **dribbling**, **layup shooting**, and **passing.** On the signal "go" the first person on each team must dribble toward the basket where they will attempt a "layup." On a make or miss the ball will be rebounded and passed (2 hand chest pass) to the next person in line, and the shooter goes to the end of the line. On every made shot the entire team counts out the number of made shots until "10" is reached. at which point the round is over and a winner is determined. Rotate teams so everyone shoots from a different angle (left or right) and at a different basket.

Tip: This game should not be played until the individual skills of : passing, dribbling, and layup shooting have been taught and practiced. Also, the game can be played where all teams compete against each other at once, or only against the team on their side of the court. In both cases, each session ends when one of the 4 teams reaches 10.

Grades: 3-5

"Basketball Kickball "

Formation: One "*kicker*" lined up behind ball.
One "*shooter*" placed near the basket the rest of the
fielding team spread out starting at the half court line
in 3 rows.
Equipment: 1 "Nerf "kickball, 4 cones (2 at half court
sideline, 2 at end line sideline), 1 home plate.

How to play:
    The **kicker** kicks the nerf ball out onto the field and starts to run outside the cones and then tags home plate. The **fielder** that catches the ball passes it to their **shooter** as fast as they can. The shooter attempts to make as many layups as they can until the kicker circles all the cones and tags Homeplate.
    The instructor will blow the whistle upon the kicker touching home plate. The fielding team scores a point for every basket made. **Continued......**

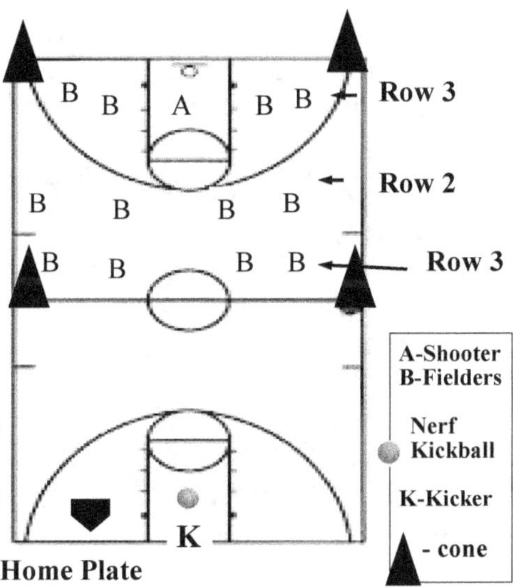

"Basketball Kickball" *continued...*   Basketball Games

Rotation: The kicker goes to the end of the line and the new kicker steps up. The fielders also rotate in any manner the instructor chooses based on class size (the traditional volleyball rotation works well). When everyone has had a chance to shoot, the teams switch. The team with the most made layups wins.

Tip:
This game is a great activity to introduce after the basketball layup game. Good passing technique and layup shooting techniques should be emphasized. The instructor can modify the height of the basket based on skill level and age of students.

"Dribble Call Ball #1"

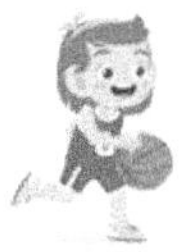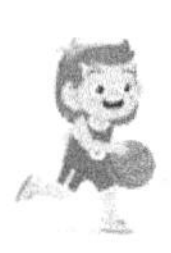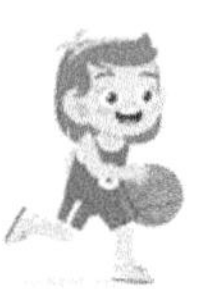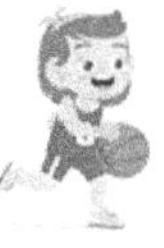

Grades: 3-5
Formation: Four (Teams) Numbered (2 teams at
half court, 2 on each sideline) (see diagram), 1 ball in front of each team.
Equipment: Four (4) Basketballs

How to Play: The Instructor calls out a number. Everyone on the 4 teams that has that number picks up the basketball in front of their team and dribbles toward the basket. Everyone continues to shoot until "3" have made a basket. All 3 teams will then receive a point . After
a missed shot, the player retrieves the ball and **must** dribble to shoot again. Once a shot is made, the student goes back to the spot they started from and places the ball down until two of the other teams make their shot. A team is awarded 1 point for each basket scored.

Tip: A shot can be attempted from anywhere, but the instructor should explain that the closer you shoot to the basket, the better chance you have to make it.

"Dribble Call Ball #2,3"
Grades: 3-5
Formation: Four teams numbered (2 teams at half court, 2 on each sideline) (see diagram on next page), 1 ball in front of each team.
Equipment: Four (4) Basketballs , (14) Poly Spots

How to Play:
    This game is played the same as "Dribble Call Ball #1 " except the players may attempt to make a **3 Point shot** or a **2 Point** shot in addition to the Lay Up **1 Point shot**.

Tips and Diagram on next page

Basketball Games

Tips on *"Dribble Call Ball"* from previous page.....

- The team losing can catch up quickly by making 3 or 2 point shots:

- Place the poly spots, depending on the classes skill.

- Example: Place the spots closer to the basket for 3rd graders, and further away for 5th graders. Also, to encourage harder shots, make a rule that a layup (1 point), cannot be attempted until they **have attempted a 2 or 3 point shot first.**

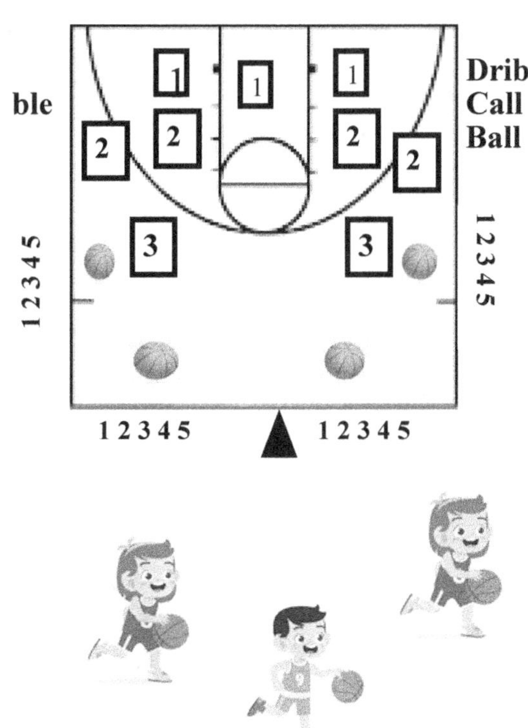

"Rotation Dribble"

Equipment: 2 Basketballs , and one Basketball Goal

How to Play:

    This game helps students to develop skills in **dribbling, shooting, rebounding,** and better accuracy in quickly passing a ball. In this game "A" is the *passing team,* and "B" is the *dribbling team.* Balls and players are arranged as shown in the diagram. The left corner player on "A" and the first player on "B" wait for the instructor's signal. Players on "A" pass the ball as indicated by the arrows; when the last team member receives the ball, they dribble (as shown) and shoot a layup. At the same time, the first "B" player dribbles the ball (as shown) ; when they complete their run, they al-so

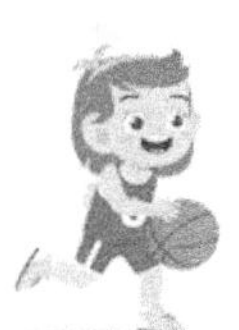
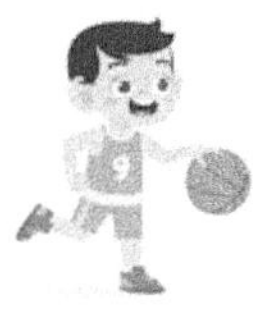
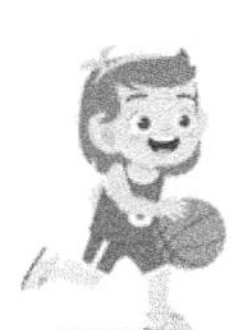

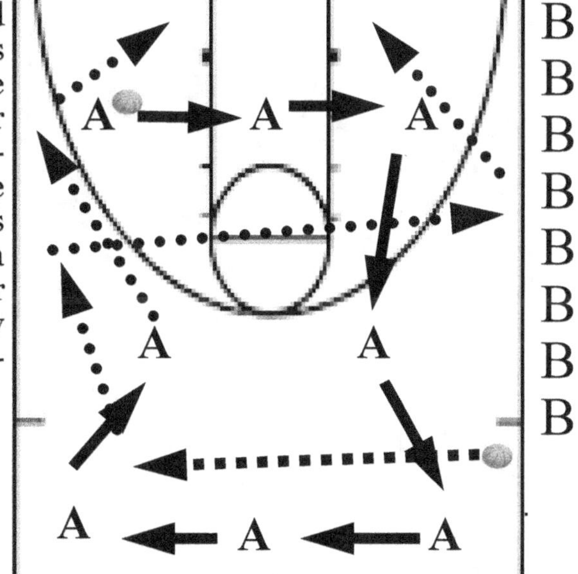

Net
&
Scooter
Games

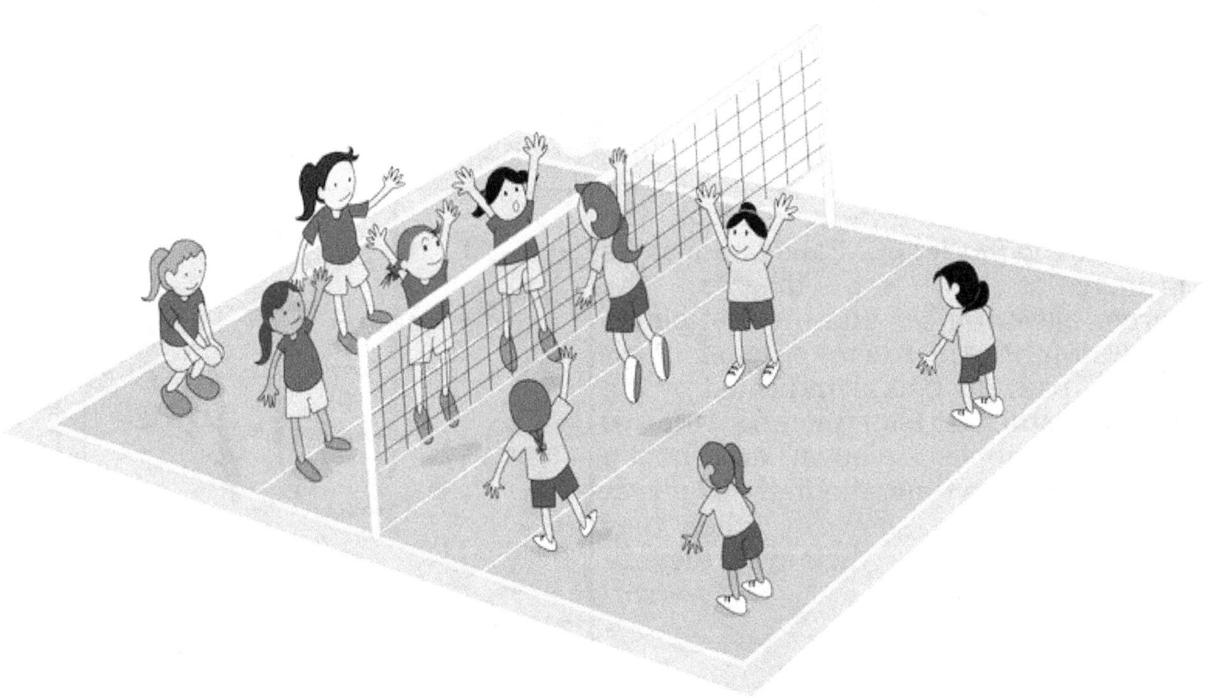

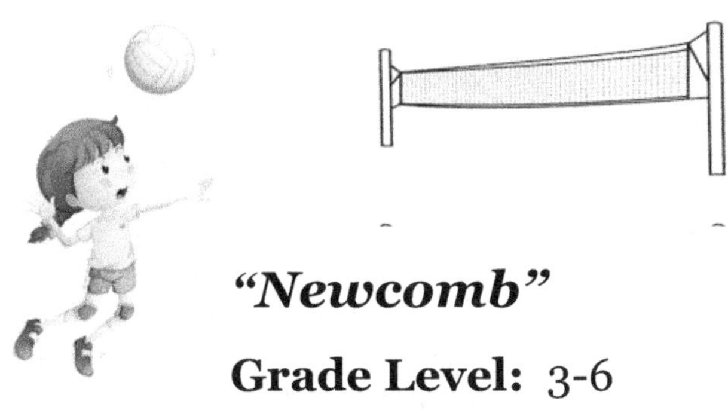

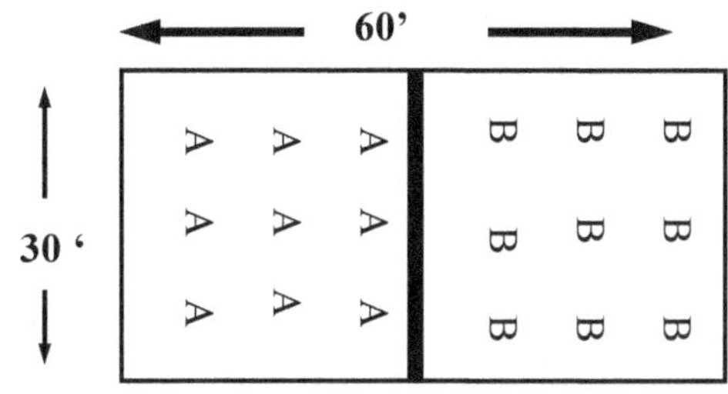

"Newcomb"

Grade Level: 3-6

Equipment: Volleyball, net,
and standards.

Formation:
Two teams, one on each side of the net.

How to Play:

The player in the back right corner (facing the net) serves the ball by throwing it over the net. Players on opposite sides of the net try to catch the ball before it hits the floor. If they are unsuccessful, the opposing team is awarded a point. If a player catches the ball, they either throw it back over the net or pass it to a teammate. Two such passes are permitted before the ball must be returned over the net. A player may not move after catching the ball. The ball is thrown back and forth over the net until it hits the floor. Each time a team scores a point it gets to serve again. A team wins when it has scored a set number of points., or when it has scored the greatest number of points within a pre-arranged time period.

Tip: Once the class becomes proficient in catching, you may want to make the game **more challenging.** If you find this to be the case, I strongly suggest that you try "double" Newcomb (some of my upper classes have played with 3 and even 4 balls). Everything is the same except that two or more balls are served at once. When the first ball hits the ground, let it stay there and continue until the second ball has dropped also, and so on until all balls have hit the ground. I strongly suggest you play "Double Newcomb +) to add even more excitement to this game. Two points are at stake each round.

"Over/Under"

Grade Level: 3-5

Equipment: 2 Volleyballs, Net,
and Standards

Formation: Two teams, one on each side of the 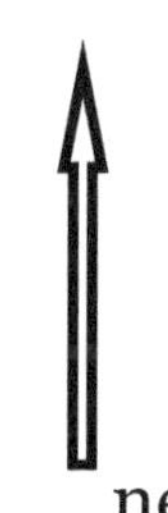 net.

How to Play: Once you have played Dodge ball and Newcomb, your classes

Continued on next page ....

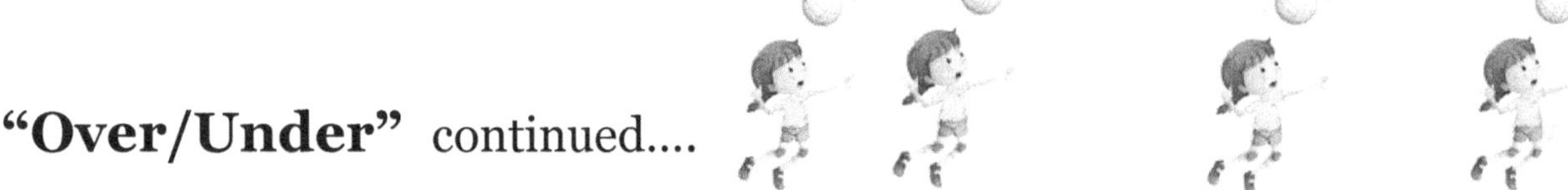

"Over/Under" continued....

are now ready to play **one of the best games I have ever used**...I call it **"Over/Under,"** and it is a combination of Newcomb and Dodgeball. Depending on how the ball is thrown, the rules of that game prevail. Any ball thrown **over** the net, use the rules of Newcomb. Any ball **under** the net use Dodgeball rules. Explain that any **over** throw can only result in points as in "Newcomb" (No elimination.) Any ball thrown **under** the net can only eliminate players as in "Dodgeball." There are no points for under throws. When a player gets hit with an under throw, they leave and go to the side of the court. When more players are eliminated, it will make it easier to score points on over throws because there will be fewer players to catch the ball.

The game is over if (10) points are scored (it doesn't matter how many players are eliminated) or if all the players on one team are eliminated regardless of how many points are scored.

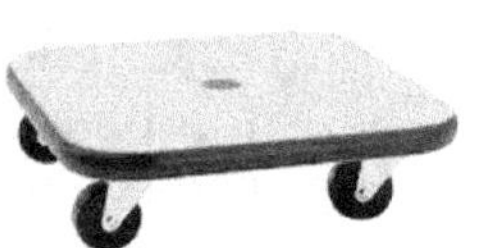

Scooter Games

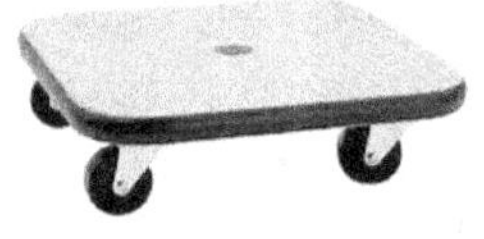

Scooters can be used for some great activities. Before we start, I explain that scooters are <u>never</u> to be stood upon. In order to stay on the scooter, I tell the students two important rules. The first is to sit in the middle and the second is not to lean. To move, dig your heels into the floor one at a time and push with your hands in the opposite direction that you want to go. Once these directions have been given, I have the students take part in the following activities:

"Scooter Drill"

Give a scooter to each student, or as many scooters that are available. For about two minutes, have the students get familiar with the scooters by moving in any direction that they want. Tell them to make sure they go in all four directions. After the time limit, blow the whistle and ask how many were able to go for two minutes without falling off?

"Scooter One Less"

Grade Level: K-5
Equipment: Enough scooters for half the class. Tennis balls (1 less than the number of kids on scooters at one time) or something similar.

Formation: Half the class sits on the scooters at one of the end lines. The other half sits behind them waiting their turn.

Continued on next page..........

Scooter Games

"Scooter One Less" continued..

How To Play:
   Throw all the balls to the opposite end of the gym. Throw **"one less"** than the number of players on scooters. On the signal from the instructor, the players attempt to retrieve a ball, and upon doing so, raise the ball in their hand and stay at that spot. When everyone has a ball, except one, blow the whistle. At that point everyone picks up the scooter and brings it back to the next person in line. Continue with the next group.

Tip: This activity shows the importance of not falling off the scooter, since it will slow you down. **For your first lesson**, the **"explanation"**, the **"Scooter drill"**, and "**Scooter One Less**" will take up an entire class period.

Tip: The second time we meet, I do scooters I play two activities: 1. Scooter Races
2. Scooter Tag

"Scooter Races"
Grade Level: K-5

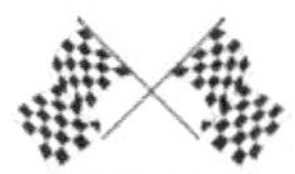

How To Play:
   Break up the class into 3 groups. On the signal, all those on the scooters must go **forward** to the end line, then **backward** to the starting line. First player back is the winner.
   Continue until all three groups have gone. When everyone has gone, have the 3 winners go against each other. I usually do this for three rotations.

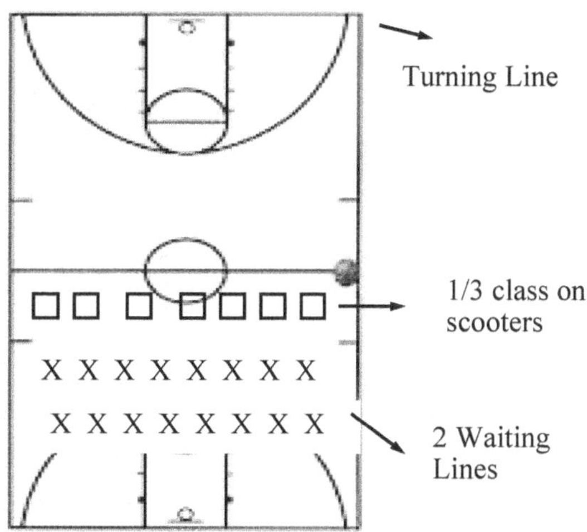

"Scooter Tag"

Grade Level: K-5
How To Play:
   If there are enough scooters, play with two teams. Otherwise, break the class up into three teams and have one group sit out and rotate in. Have the teams start behind the sidelines. Designate one team as the "taggers" and the other team as those trying to set across the other line. On the signal "go" the team that is attempting to score may go in any direction they would like to try to get across before being tagged. (Important: a player must be tagged with a hand, not a leg).

Continued.....

Scooter Games

Scooter Tag Diag.

"Scooter Tag" *continued...*

The tagging team members attempt to tag play-ers before they cross the opposite sideline.
Once tagged, a student must stop moving and raise their hand until the whistle blows end-ing the session. If any player, tagged or those at-tempting to tag, falls off of their scooter, the pen-alty is to sit on the floor until the whistle is blown.
Score 1 point for everyone who successful-ly crosses the line and switch roles to continue the round.

Tip: A tagger may tag more than one opponent.

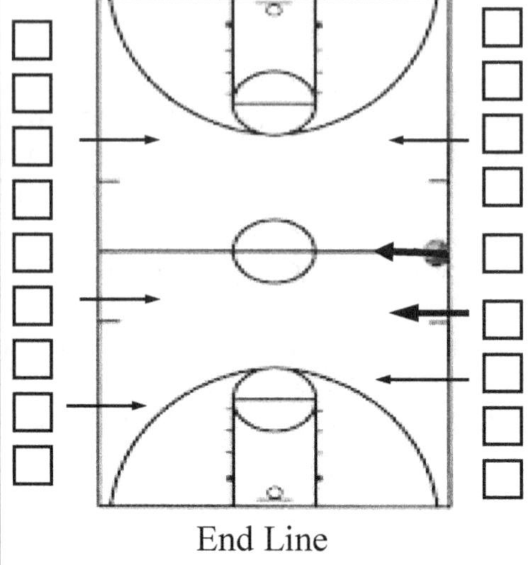

"Scooter Box Ball"

Grade Level: 3-5

Formation: Two teams line up on scooters behind the side line. Partners are sitting next to each other. The partners decide who is the "chaser" and who is the "thrower." (They will switch during next round).

Equipment: Scooters for every student, balls (whiffle balls or tennis balls work great). Instructor throws out as many balls as possible. I have done this with up to 100 balls, 50 at each end.

Rules:
No player, chaser or thrower may have more than 1 ball in their hand at a time. Throwers attempting to throw the ball into their team's container **may not** enter the cen-ter circle with their feet or scooter.

How To Play:

On the signal, the **"chasers"** head down toward where the balls are, while the **"throwers"** position themselves around the circle. When a chaser has a ball, they throw it to their throwing partner, who attempts to throw it into the correct container. Continue the process until there are no more balls left. When there are no more balls left, the whistle blows. At this point all the players pick up their scooter and return them to the original spots. Count the balls in both containers and either declare a winner or keep a cumulative score each round for the entire class period. The game continues with the throwers and catchers changing places.

Continued.....

"Scooter Box Ball" continued...   Scooter Games

Tips:

- Any ball that gets stuck in the circle must stay, the teacher may take them out of the circle during the game.
- Whatever side of the half-court the players start on, is the side they must stay on. Do not allow anyone to cross half court.
- Once a thrower has a ball, they cannot be blocked by an opposing player.
- Any ball thrown by a "chaser" to a "thrower" may be intercepted.

Scooter Box Ball Starting Positions   **Possible Positions Once Game Starts**

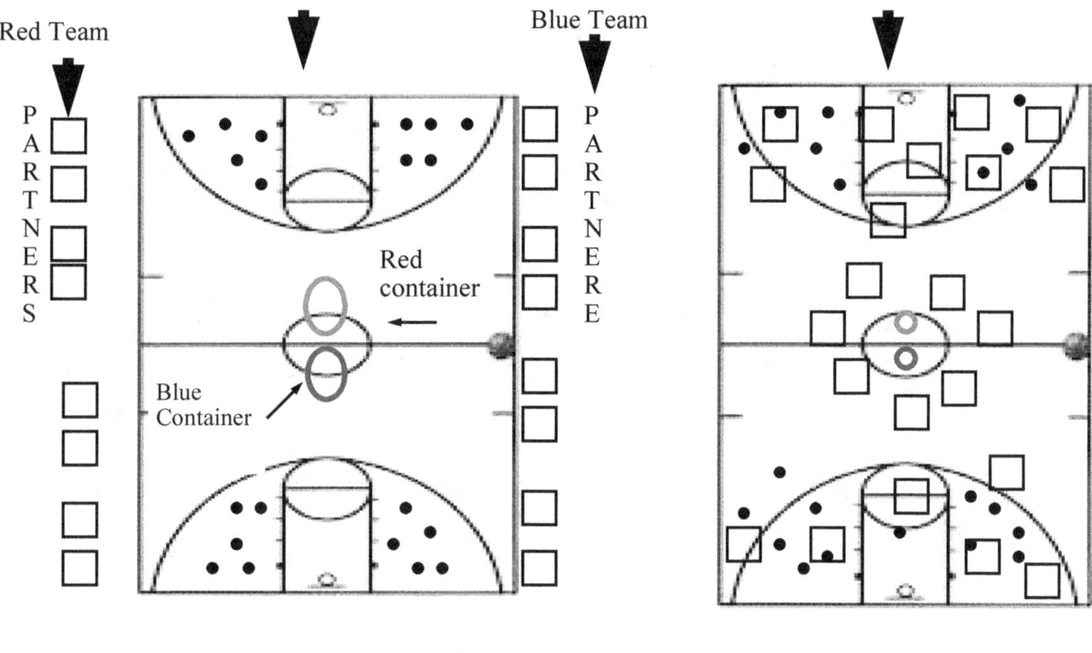

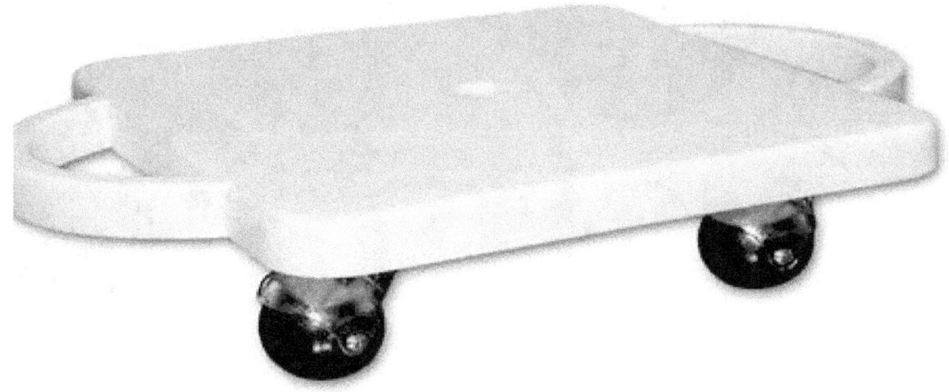

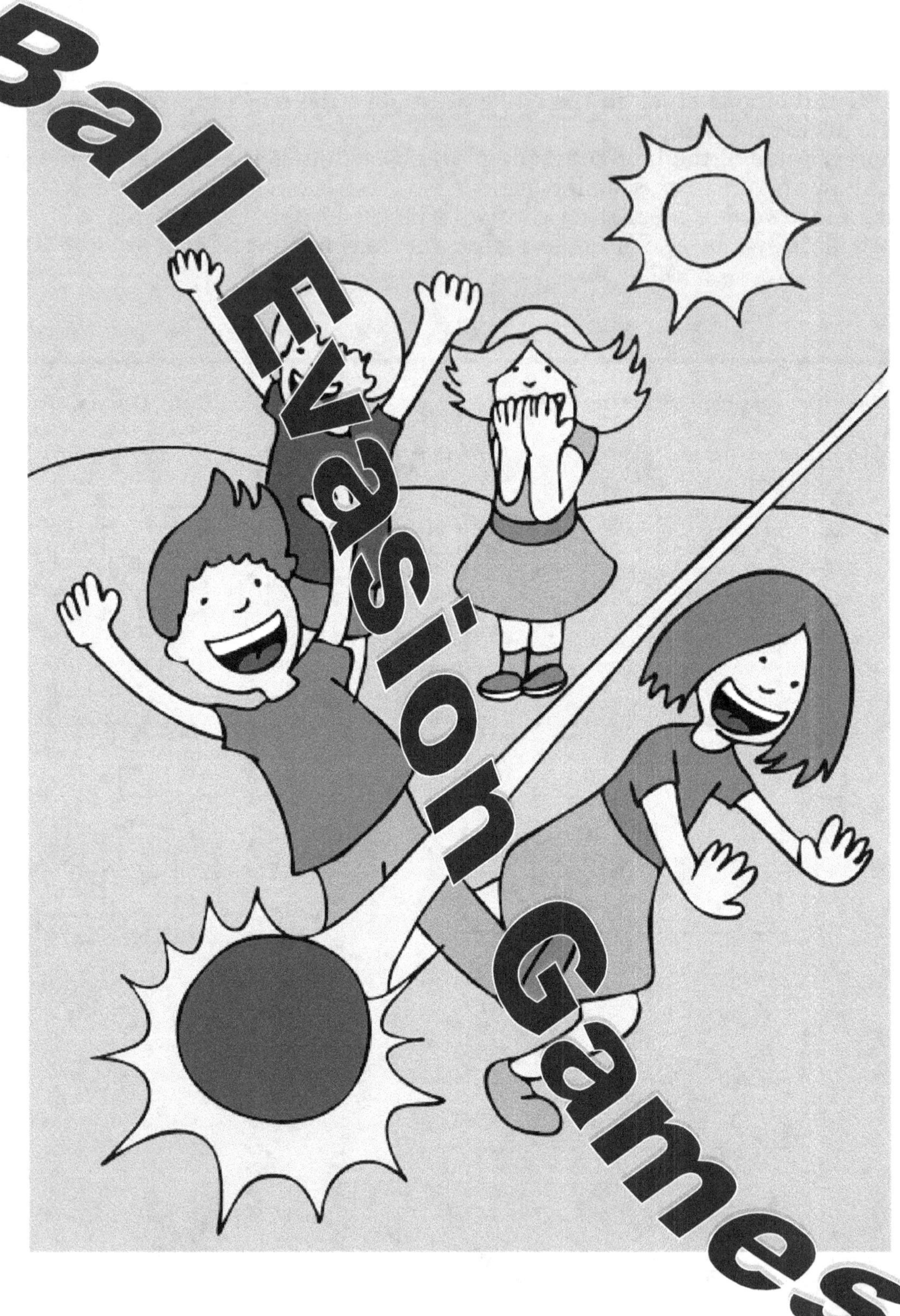

Ball Evasion Games

Ball Evasion Games

Dodgeball, (ball evasion) is an activity that students of all ages love. **Before you start your "ball evasion" unit, you should choose balls that are lightweight.** I strongly disapprove of rubber playground balls. Rules should be established, and strictly adhered to. You must demand that **all balls are to be thrown below the waist.** Lightweight balls are used because unfortunately, the throwing skills of children this age, are not always accurate.

How to Play

(Level 1)

The Instructor calls out either "Red" "Yellow" or "Blue". All those sitting in that colored hoop stand up with their ball. The first way to play this game is **"no elimination".**

Students try to hit anyone they can with their ball (no tagging with the ball, it must be thrown). After they throw their ball, they may go find any ball that is on the ground to use to hit someone else. Let the game go for about 1 minute. When the whistle blows, everyone goes and gets any color ball and they all go back to their original hoop. Play until all colored hoops have had a turn.

Have the students try to remember how many targets (students) they hit and ask them when they get back. Because there is no elimination, explain: "The closer you get to your target, the better chance you will have to hit someone.

(Level 2):

This is an elimination game. Everything is the same except this time when you are hit, you must sit at that spot. Play continues until only 1 player is left. After all 3 colors are called the instructor calls the winner from each color to come out and play for the championship. Because this is an elimination game you explain that you might want to "sneak up" on someone, and get really close before you throw your ball. Teacher can call more than 1 color to add variety.

"Color Hoop Ball"

Grades PK-2
Formation: See Diagram.
Equipment: Each student sits in a colored hoop with a ball. The ball doesn't have to be the same color as the hoop, but it can be.

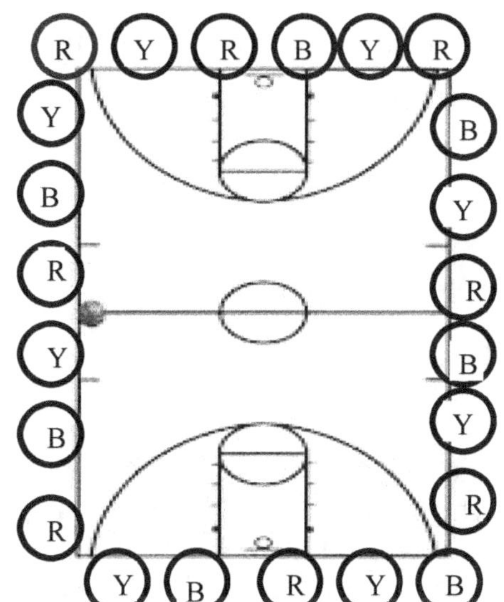

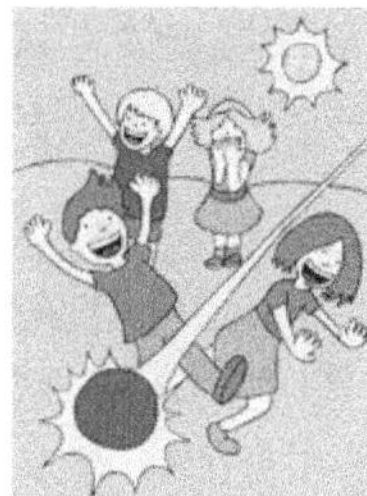

"Four Team Smush"

Ball Evasion Games

Grades: 2-5
Formation: Each team is numbered and sits behind their team's ball.
Equipment: A different colored ball for each team.

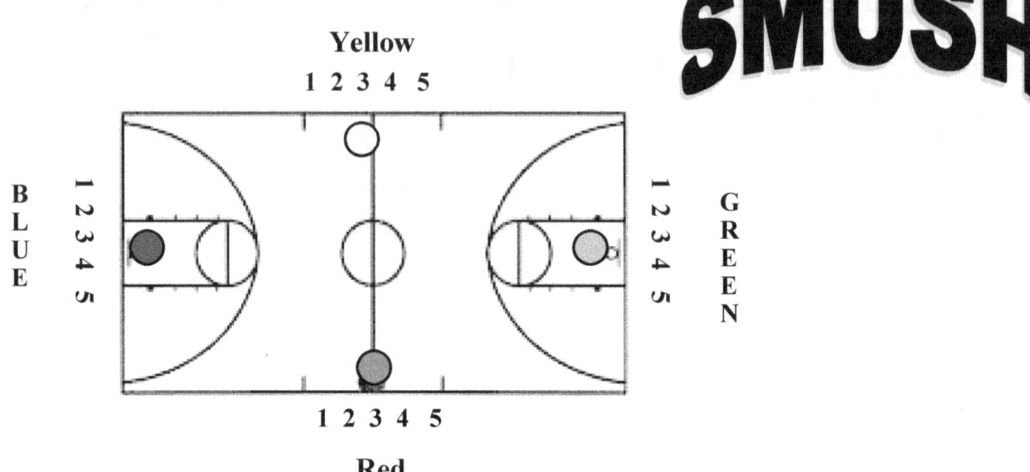

How to Play:
The instructor calls out a number. The person who has that number picks up the ball. The four that are playing are trying to be the **last one left**." In this game you can only throw your team's color ball.

Tip: Depending on how many different color balls you have, you may play with more than 4 teams. Note: The more the better.

"Shadow Dodgeball"

Grade Level: All   "A favorite of all grade levels"

How to Play:
  This takes "Smush" to a new level! Everything is the same as "4 Team Smush" except two numbers are called at once. Obviously only one player can pick up the ball. The teammate without the ball becomes the "Shadow". Instruct them to stay as close behind the player with the ball as possible and do everything they do (become their shadow). If the player with the ball gets hit, get the ball to your "shadow" before you sit. Because two numbers are called there is an opportunity to score 2 points in each round.

Tip: Explain to students that they should stay as close to their teammate as possible when he has the ball. When neither of the teammates have the ball (because it has been thrown), separate and try to recover your team's ball before you get hit. Then get your shadow back.

" Battle Royale"

Ball Evasion Games

Grades 2-5
Formation: 4 Teams forming a square with each team covering 1/4 of a half Court.

How to Play: One player from each team starts by moving toward the foul line, with their back to their team. One ball is given to one player on each of the 4 teams. The object of the game is to be the last player who has not been hit. When a player gets hit, they sit at the spot where they were hit.

To start the game, instruct the outside people who have a ball to be careful not to hit their own player which will cause them to be out. The rules are quite simple. The players on the outside cannot step over the lines either by throwing or catching a ball. The inside people can run anywhere they want to avoid being hit except to step outside the lines.

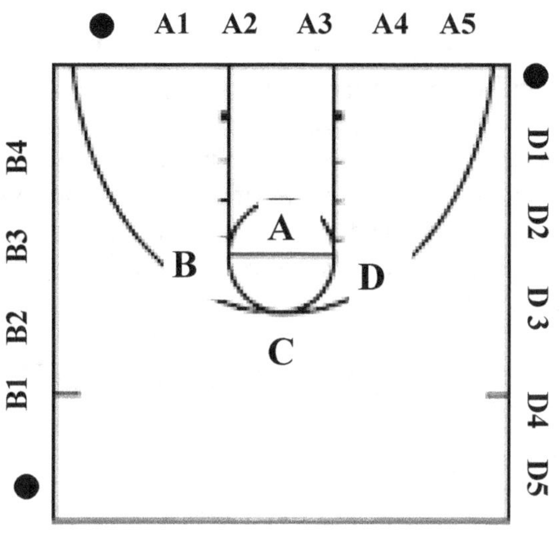

This next part makes the game very challenging:

Instruct the players who start inside the square to: **#1** Avoid any balls that are thrown, but at the same time, you are allowed to pick up any thrown ball that stays inside the lines. With a ball in hand, they may chase any player and attempt to throw the ball and hit them (tagging with a ball is not allowed). Continue play until one person is left and award that team a point.

Rotation: The 4 players in the square replace a member of their team on the sideline, who then steps into the middle to start a new round.

" Hoop Maze"

Hoop Maze

Grades K-5

Formation:
- "Running Team" - lined up behind end line.

- "Throwing Team" - scattered around with each player standing in a hoop with a ball .

**A -Throwers
Each with a
ball, standing
in hoops**

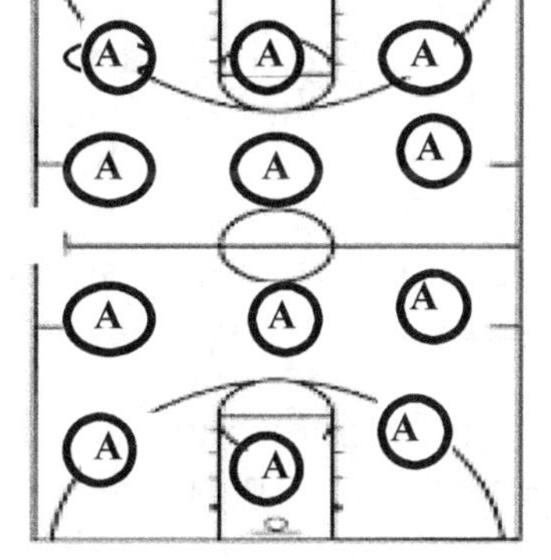

Continued on next page.......... **X Runners**

" Hoop Maze" continued

Ball Evasion Games

How to Play:

On the signal "go" all the "runners" attempt to cross to the opposite end line without getting hit with a ball. If a runner is hit , they must stop and raise their hand until the round is completed.

Tip: Throwers may throw another ball if they can secure one without stepping out of their hoop. Instruct runners to stay away from hoops that still have a ball, while running close to hoops that have no ball.   Since runners may wait until no balls are in the hoops, you may want to set a time limit to get across the opposite end line. If a runner is unable to get to the other side before the time limit is up, they are considered hit.

To start the next round, have all runners who were hit go to the other side and have all hoop players retrieve a ball. After a certain number of rounds switch the runners and the throwers.

" Field Dodgeball"

Grades 2-5

Equipment: 1 Nerf dodgeball, 5 cones

Formation:
1 runner starts at the starting line (When coming back it is the finish line) between the two cones. The fielding team is spread out in the field in 3 rows (right, center, left). The last person on the left starts with a ball.

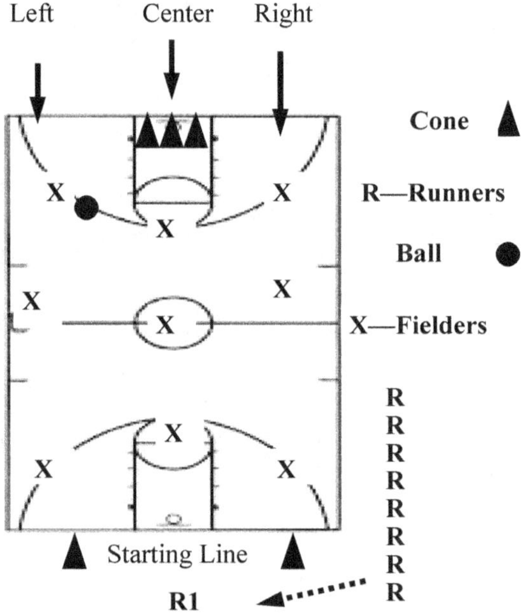

How to Play:
On the signal "go" the runner attempts to work their way down the court, run around the 3 cones at the end of the gym, and tries to get back to the finish line without getting hit with the ball.

The fielding team attempts to hit the runner before they get back. Since the runner will run away from the person with the ball, passing to a teammate closer to the runner should be emphasized. 1 point is scored for each successful run.

Rules: The fielders have 2 simple rules: **1:** You cannot hold the ball in your hands longer than 3 seconds, and **2:** You are not allowed to run with the ball to hit the runner. On an errant pass you are allowed to run to to get the ball, but you must pass or throw from that point.

The runners simply have 1 rule: You must run around the cones at the end of the gym, and cross the finish line <u>between</u> the two cones.

Continued........

Ball Evasion Games

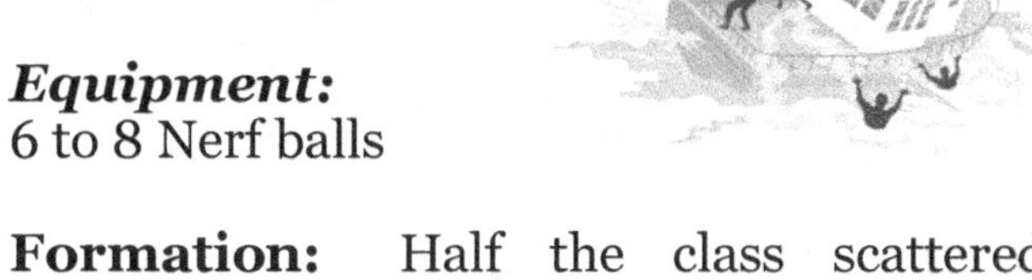

"Field Dodgeball" continued...

Tip: Emphasize teamwork to the fielders. A fielder from the left side should not attempt to hit the runner on the right side. A pass to a teammate on the right side will make an easier hit possible.

Rotation: Runner goes to end of running line and a new runner steps in. Fielders rotate clockwise so that they are changing to a new position with each runner. Once your class has the basics for this game, try using multiple runners at one time. (We have actually played this with as many as 6 runners at a time). When using multiple runners, all runners who get hit must stop and raise their hand until the round is over.

"Free For All Survivor"

Grades: K-5

Equipment:
6 to 8 Nerf balls

Formation: Half the class scattered around the gym, the other half waits out of bounds.

How to Play:

Once the group is scattered around the gym, the teacher throws a ball anywhere onto the court. Whoever gets the ball, attempts to hit anyone (you may run and get as close as you can to your target). Once the ball is thrown, anyone may pick it up. When a player gets hit they sit at that spot.

The teacher throws out balls every few seconds so players must be aware of the extra balls. Play until one (1) is left and then switch groups. This is a great warm-up activity. I usually play 2 rounds of boys, then 2 rounds of girls. The final round consists of the 4 winners who each go to a corner of the gym and play until an overall

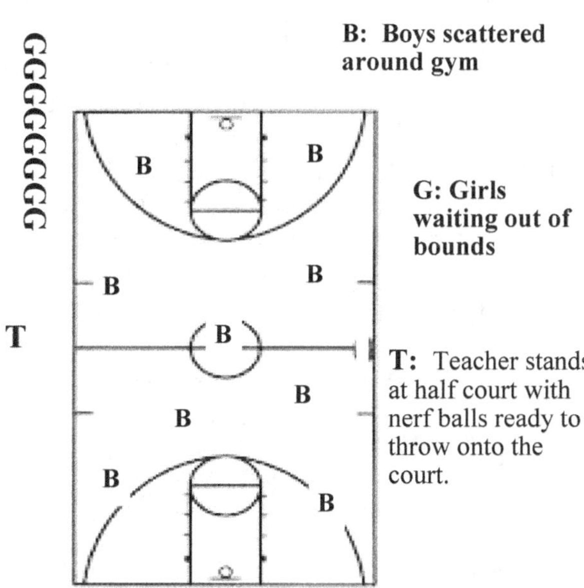

winner is left.

Rules: Once you throw a ball, anyone can pick it up, and the thrower may get any ball that they can. Only 1 ball may be held at a time.

Because of the popularity of the TV show, I call this game "Survivor" The kids really get excited when I use that name!!

" Traitor "   Ball Evasion Games

Grades: *3-5*

Equipment:
8 to 10 Balls, each team getting half the balls.

Formation: Team "A" scatters on half the court. Team "B" scatters on the other half. One player from "A" is the traitor, and they go to the B side and must stay in the foul circle.. The same with the "B" team traitor. No player from either team may cross the 1/2 court line or enter the traitor's circle. Players are

How to Play: No player from either team may cross the 1/2 court line or enter the traitor's circle. Players are allowed to cross the sidelines and end line only to retrieve a ball.

Team "A" attempts to eliminate the **"B" team** and vice versa. Game continues until all players on one team are eliminated, or set a time limit with the team having the most players still in the game when time is up winning.

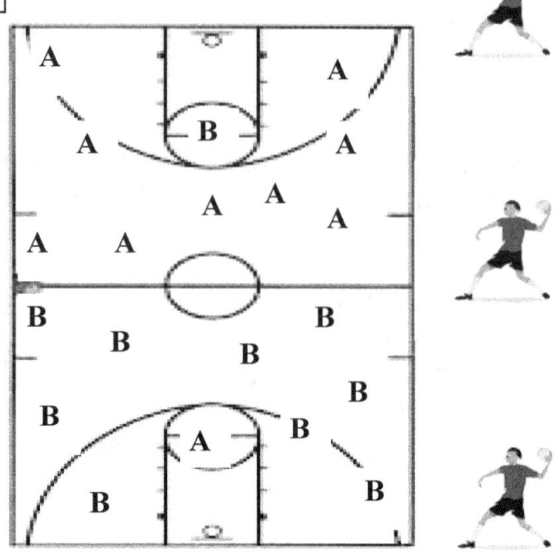

Tip: Explain to the teams that if they can't hit someone because they are too far away, pass it to their traitor, and they will have a better chance. If played strategically, most players will be eliminated by the traitor. Once a team is eliminated, choose new "traitors" and continue.

"Medic"

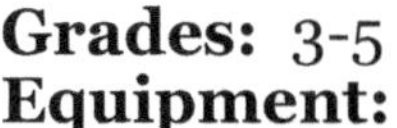

Grades: 3-5
Equipment:
2 Scooters. And 8 to 10 balls, each team getting half the balls to start.

Formation: Team "A" scatters on half the court. Team "B" scatters on the other half. One member of team A and B, stands behind the end line of their team holding a scooter. They are the **"MEDICS"**

How to Play: Regular dodgeball rules apply, but players who get eliminated, may be "rescued" and brought back into the game. The player who gets hit sits down at that spot. The "medic" runs to that player and places the "ambulance" (scooter) down and the "injured" player sits on the scooter facing the "hospital" (area behind his end line). The medic gently places a hand on their back and helps guide the player to the "hospital zone". Once there, the player may re-enter the game. Set a time limit, and when the time is up blow the whistle. Count all the players who are still standing. The team with the most standing wins. Anyone on a scooter when the whistle blows **does not count.**
Tip: sometimes its fun to have two medics on each team .

" Traitor Medic"

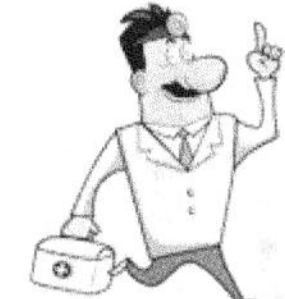

Ball Evasion Games

Grades: 3-5

Equipment:
4 scooters, and 8 to 10 balls, each team getting half the balls.

Formation: Team "A" scatters on half the court. Team "B" scatters on the other half. One player from "A" is the traitor, and they go to the B side and must stay in the foul circle.. The same with the "B" team traitor. No player from either team may cross the 1/2 court line or enter the traitor's circle. In addition 2 players from each team are designated as "medics" and given scooters. They line up behind their teams end line just as they do in the game "medic."

How to Play: Once your class has played "Traitor" , then "Medic", combine the two games to play one of the most fast moving, exciting games, there is. Same rules as used for "medic" and "traitor". I would definitely use 2 medics, since players will be getting hit quickly because of the traitor. Play either by a specific time (2 minutes is good) or until all members of one team have been eliminated. Start the next game with new "medics" and also new "traitors."

"Prisoner Dodgeball "

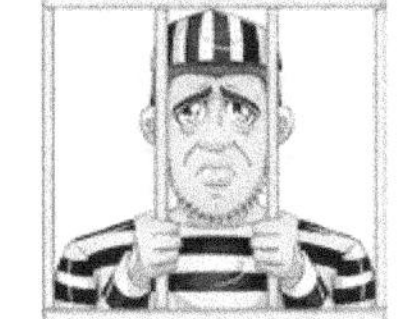

Grades: 3-5
Equipment:
8 to 10 Nerf Balls (half to each team)

Formation: The **A** team is scattered on half the court, and the **B** team on the other. One player from each team starts in their team's "prison area."

How to Play:
    This is a unique dodgeball game because no one is ever permanently eliminated. When a player is hit, they leave via the sideline (they do not cross the half court line) and proceed to their prison area where they can still throw balls at the other team members.

    The object of the game is for one team to put their opponents entire team in prison. The first team to accomplish this is the winner.

Note:
1. **Prisoners are not allowed to cross the end line to retrieve a ball, and vice versa.**
2. **No one is allowed to cross the half court line to retrieve a ball.**

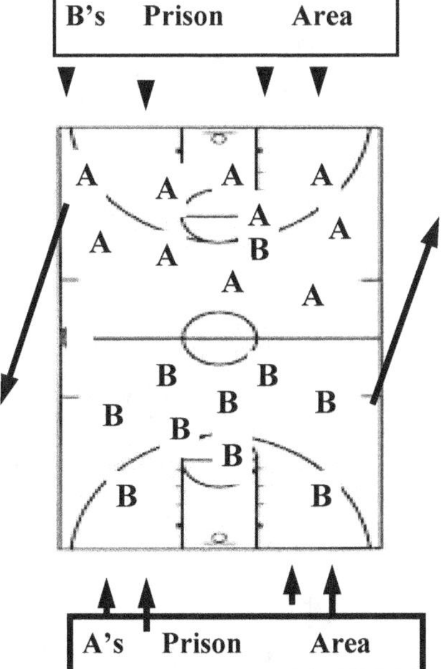

Tip: Encourage players to help free prisoners by passing them the ball.

Skill Components

Movements 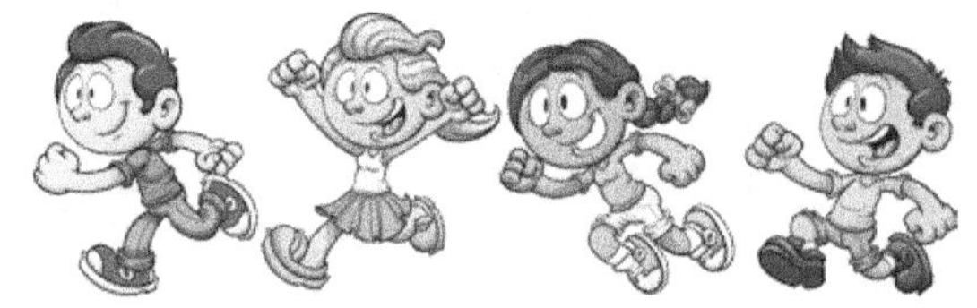

Throwing 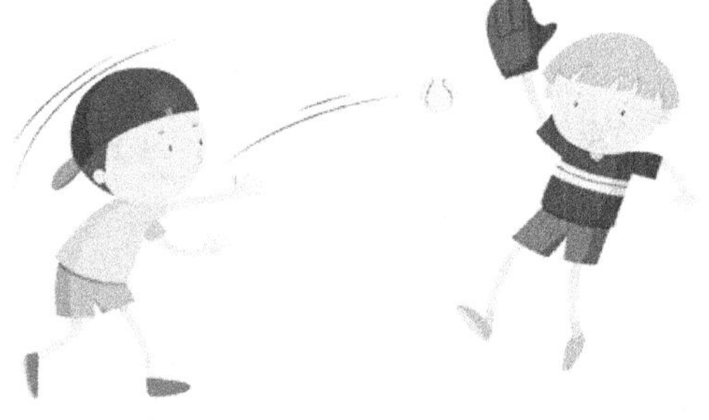

Catching

Kicking 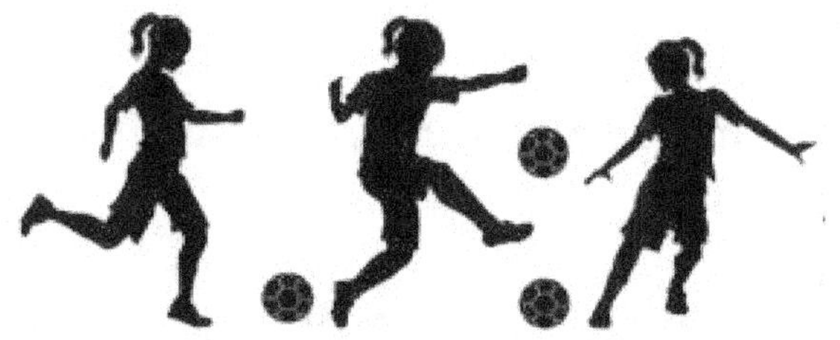

Movement

The components of each skill represent a sampling of the many aspects that each skill requires for mastery. The reader is encouraged to have a general conception of the critical parts of each skill and add or subtract from this list to meet your needs. If necessary, it is possible to evaluate student competency by using all or some of these components.

Walking

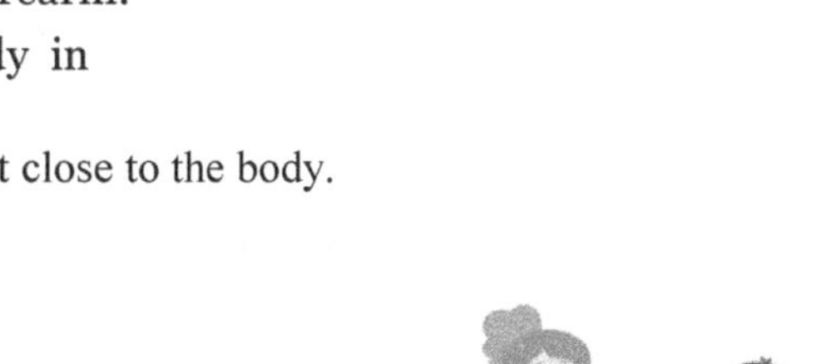

- Body weight directly over the feet.
- Back straight and relaxed.
- Shoulders back
- Swing legs from the hip.
- Bend the knee of the foot clearing the floor.
- Push off the rear foot.
- Touch the back of the forward foot first, then the ball of foot as you transfer weight to the toes.
- Walk toes pointed straight ahead. Your arms should swing freely back and forth opposite your foot movement.

Running

- Place left foot in advance of the right and lean slightly forward as you move.
- Form a 90 degree angle between the upper arm and forearm.
- Arms should swing back and forward close to your body in opposite direction of leg movement.
- Do not swing arms from side to side, they should be kept close to the body.
- Drive knees up high as close to waist high as possible.
- Keep your hands closed (fingers together).

Hopping

- Stand on one foot.
- Bend one leg at the knee and stand on one foot.
- Spring up and down on the foot touching the ground.
- Keep your body balanced .

Jumping

- Stand with both feet together about shoulder width.
- Springing from the toes, jump forward into the air driving your arms upward.
- Land balanced with both feet in the starting position
- Bend your knees slightly to absorb the bounce when you land.

Galloping

- Place one foot forward.
- Bring rear foot up to heel of the front foot.
- Step again with the forward foot, and repeat.

Sliding

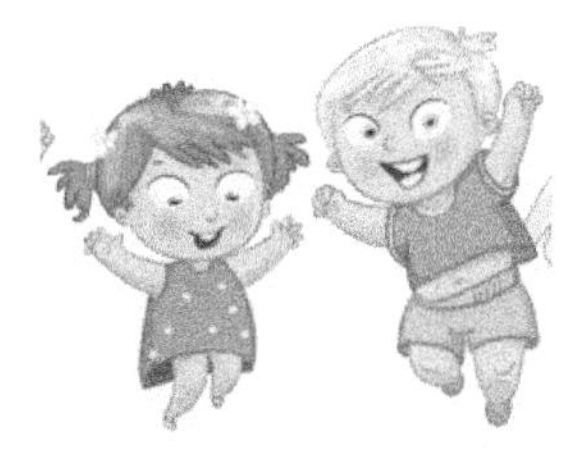

- Step sideward to the right with the right foot.
- Slide or draw the left foot to the side of the right foot.
- Shift body weight to the left foot.
- Step again with the right foot and repeat.
- Keep your head up to help your balance

Movement Skills Continued.......

<u>Skipping</u>

- The action is a step, hop.
- Step forward with either foot.
- Hop in the air on this foot.
- The arms aid in getting height and balance.
- Now, step forward with the opposite foot and repeat the action of a step, hop.

Throwing Skills (Playground ball)

Two Hand Underhand Throw

- Stand with both feet shoulders width apart, knees bent slightly.
- Hold the ball with the fingertips at each side.
- Slowly bring the ball down and back between the knees, arms extended.
- Swing the arms in a forward motion, straighten the legs as you release the ball, and follow through.

Two Hand Shoulder Throw

- Stand sideways, feet shoulder width apart, front foot pointed slightly left of your target (for right handers).
- Hold the ball with the fingertips on each side.
- Bring the ball above and slightly behind the rear shoulder using both hands.
- Propel the arms forward toward the target, and release the ball in the direction of the target with your dominant hand, follow through.

Throwing Skills (Small balls)

One Hand Overhand Throw

- Turn sideways, non-throwing hand shoulder facing the target.
- Keep your elbow at a 45 degree angle (Higher than the shoulder)
- Step slightly to the left of target (for right hand throwers)
- Swing your hips, and release ball simultaneously, follow through.

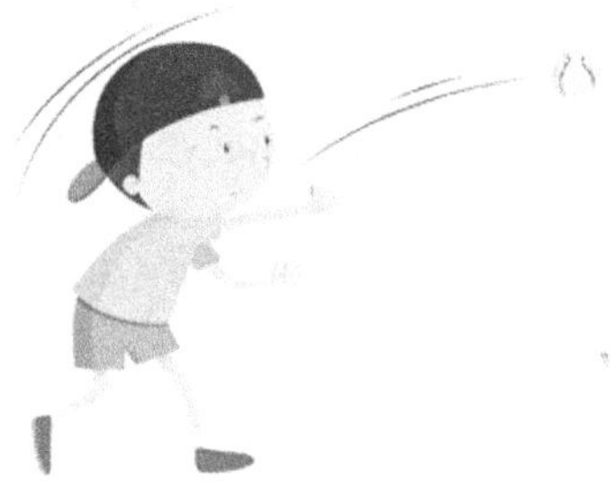

One Hand Underhand Throw

- Face your target.
- Step with your opposite foot slightly to the left of target (For right handers).
- Use a pendulum arm motion with the arm you are throwing with (like you are rolling a ball).
- Follow through.

Catching Skills

- Place your body in line with the ball (One foot slightly in front of the other, feet shoulder width apart).
- Keep your eyes on the ball.
- Hands reach out to meet the ball.
- Keep your fingers relaxed and slightly cupped.
- Reach for ball and catch with two hands (if ball arrives above waist "hands up", below waist "hands down." Do not flinch or blink.
- Watch the ball go into your hands and squeeze ball firmly to catch it.
- Bend elbows and knees slightly as you catch ball to soften impact.

Kicking Skills

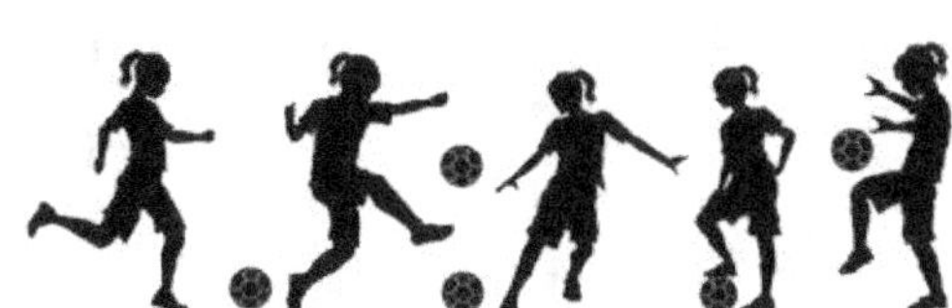

Basic Soccer Kick

- Keep your eyes on the part of the ball to be kicked.
- The lower the point of contact by the foot on the ball, the more elevation the kick will have. Adjust to your need.
- Maintain good body balance using your legs and feet.
- To improve accuracy, the foot should move directly through the ball on a path in line with the target.
- Most kicking skills should be developed in both the right and left foot.
- Kicking with the toe as in the straight-on football kickoff has little value in the game of soccer.

Instep Kick

- The instep kick is the basic soccer kick. The kicker is two or three steps bock of the ball at an angle.
- The non-kicking foot is placed alongside the ball 6 to 8 inches away with the kicking leg cocked for the kick.
- Just before contact, the kicking foot is locked so that the toe is down.
- Contact is made with the lower part of the shoe around the lower laces, with good forward snap of the lower leg at the knee. A normal follow through is desirable.
- A variation of this kick is made with the inside of the foot just above the big toe to provide a kind of easy loft shot to elevate the ball.

Inside Foot Kick

- This kick is generally used for accurate passing, but can be used for dribbling and shooting.
- The non kicking foot is drawn back, the toe is turned out.
- During the kick the toe remains turned out so the inside of the foot is perpendicular to the line of flight.
- The sole is kept parallel to the ground. The distance of the kick determines the amount of follow through.

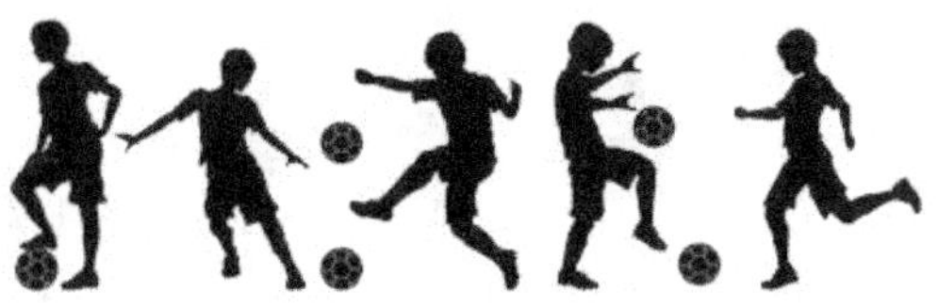

Attention All

- Superintendents
- Principals
- Department Chairs
- Head Counselors

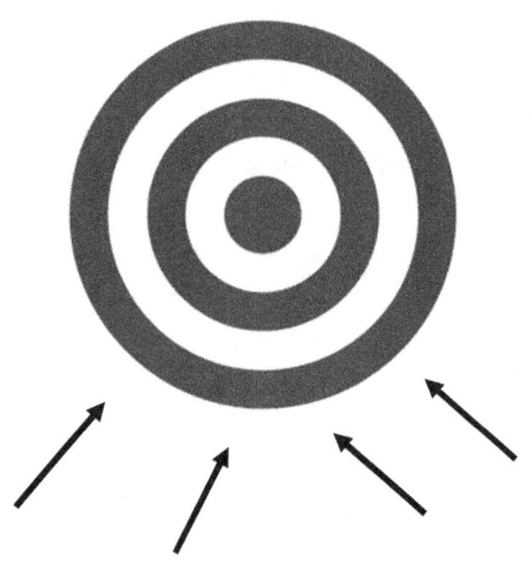

Target
Your Professional Development Day To Meet the Needs of Your Physical Education Staff!

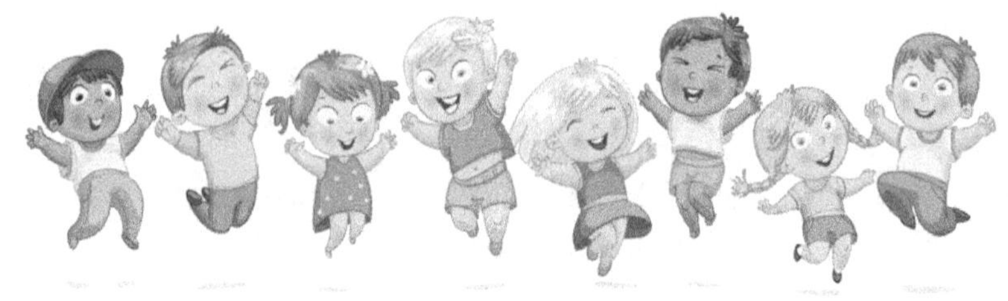

Add Excitement and Purpose To Your Next "Professional Development Day"

Make your next "Professional Development Day" a worthwhile experience for your Physical Education Teachers, Elementary Classroom Teachers with Physical Education Responsibilities, and Camp Counselors.

Find out how you can bring Tom and Jim to your district for a fraction of the cost your are now paying for programs that have no relevance to your Physical Education Staff.

Half or full day programs can be tailored to the individual needs of your staff with our "hands on" workshop featuring several of the activities and featured in this publication.

For more information email us at:

jweagan@yahoo.com
or
tcaione@comcast.net

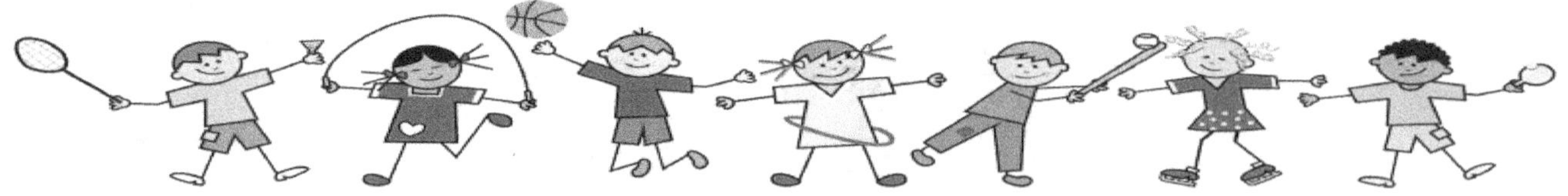

Equipment List

The supplies and equipment listed below contain a complete list of what you will need to present every game in this publication to your students. It also provides you with an excellent guide to assist you with your budget preparation.

30" Multicolor hoops	3 dozen (red, yellow, blue)
Fun balls (baseball size)	8 dozen
Tennis balls	1 dozen
12 inch rubber cones	1 dozen
Numbered cone collars	1 dozen (numbered: 1 thru 12)
6 inch playground balls	30
9 inch Poly spots	2 dozen
"Uncoated " 6 inch foam balls	1 dozen
"Training "volleyballs	4
8 and 1/4 inch "coated" kick balls	5 (1 red, 1 yellow, 3 blue)
Pinnies various colors	2 dozen
Hula hoop storage bag	2
5" x 5" bean bags (various colors)	2 dozen
Foam soccer balls	3
Bowling pins	2 Dozen
Scooters	2 dozen "(12 "blue" 12 "yellow")
Rubber bases	1 set of 4
Flip scoreboard	1
Volleyball net and standards	1 Set
Junior size basketballs	4

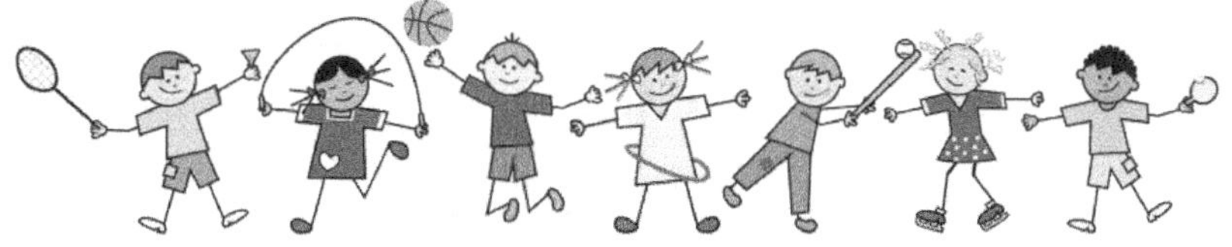

Notes:

The following pages contain space for you to list notes regarding each activity. This might be a good place to jot down specific things about each game that you might want to remember the next time you present it to your students. Examples of this could be something about your equipment or supply needs, how the children enjoyed the game, and modifications that you might make, etc. This will allow you to keep all information about these games in one place.

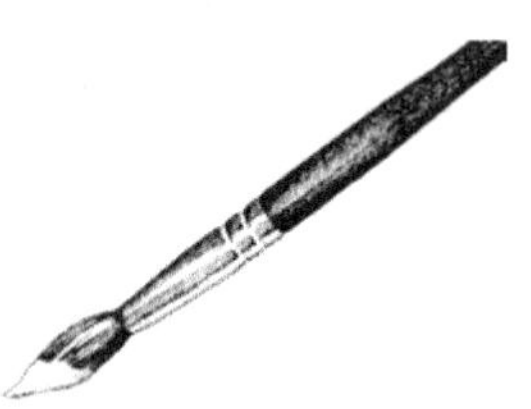 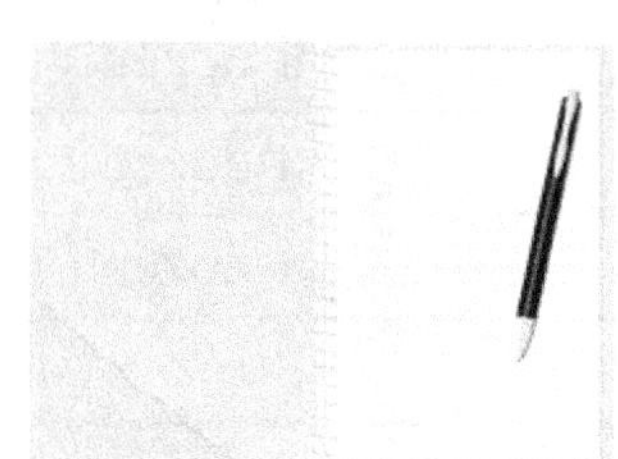 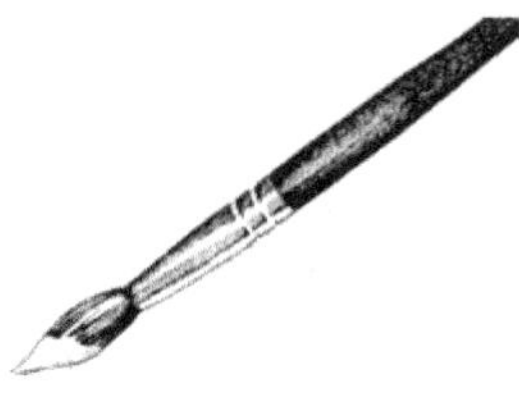

Squirrels In The Trees

Squirrels In A Tree" (Gathering Nuts)

"Bonus Ball"

"Forest Lookout"

"Whistle Mixer"

"Touchdown"

"Steal The Bacon"

"Bird Catcher"

"Coconut Tree"

"Mickey Mouse"

Man From Mars

Hoop Color Tag

Ghostbuster Tag

Bean Bag Change

Double Bean Bag Change

Water Sprite

Club Snatch

Red, Yellow. Blue Kickball

Kickball 1,2,3

Mystery Kickball

Alaskan Kickball

Line Soccer

Knockdown Rotational Kickball

Kick Pin Defense

Kick Pin Kickball

Sock It To Me

Throw and Go

Double Trouble

Stop Thief

Pin Pass

Double Pin Pass

Guard The Castle

Pin Bombardment

End Ball

Freedom Ball

Basketball Target Throw

Water Sprite With A Ball

Guard The Castle Full Court

Progressive Bowling

Alley Ball

4 Team Pinball

Castle Ball

Castle Knockdown

Castle Knockdown Rebuild

Basketball Lay Ups

Basketball Kickball

Dribble Call Ball #1

Dribble Call Ball #2

Dribble Call Ball #3

Rotation Dribble

Newcomb

Over/Under

Scooter Drill

Scooter "One Less

Scooter Races

Scooter Tag

Scooter Box Ball

Color Hoop Ball

Four Team Smush

Shadow Dodgeball

Battle Royale

Hoop Maze

Field Dodgeball

Free For All "Survivor"

Traitor

Medic

Traitor Medic

Prisoner Dodgeball

Additional Notes